MM DCPL0000181275

D0496494

OFF THE RAILS
LOVE YOUR LOOK

Sonya Lennon & Brendan Courtney

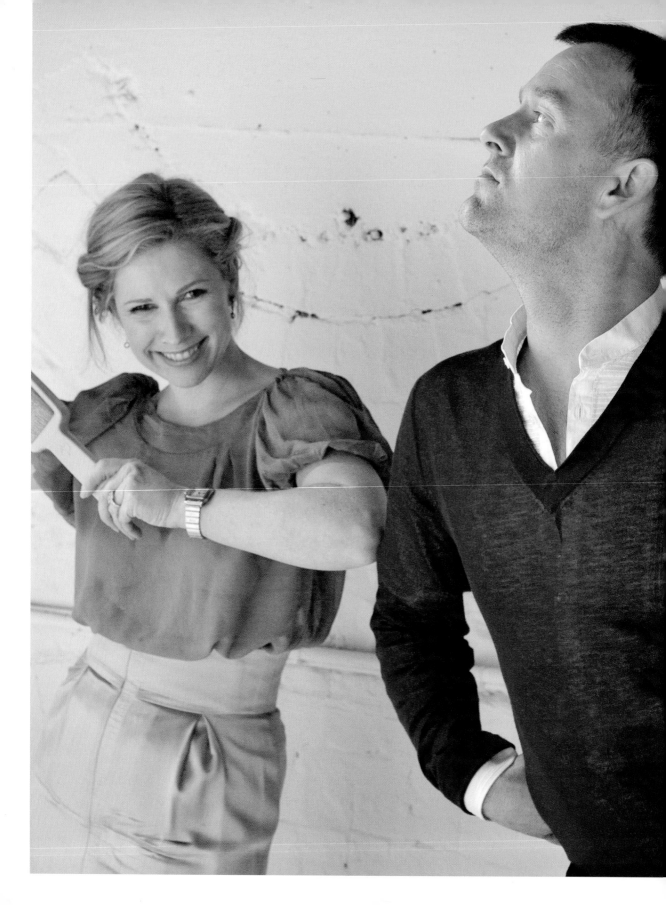

OFF THE RAILS
LOVE YOUR LOOK

Sonya Lennon & Brendan Courtney

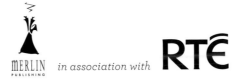

MERLIN
PUBLISHING

in association with RTÉ

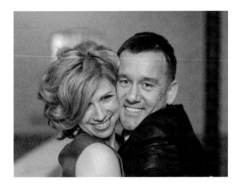

We would like to dedicate this book to all the women, both on TV and in the pages of this book, whom we have had the honour of working with. You are a truly inspirational group of women. *Sonya & Brendan*

Clothes are never a matter of pure and simple aesthetics: there are too many intimate feelings involved. Clothes play such an important role in the delicate business of self-expression, that it seems impossible to discuss objectively at any length.
ELIZABETH BOWEN, 1899 – 1973 (Irish writer and doyen of fabulousness!)

First published in 2009 by:

Merlin Publishing
Newmarket Hall, Cork Street,
Dublin 8, Ireland

T +353 1 4535866
F +353 1 4535930
E publishing@merlin.ie

www.merlinwolfhound.com

Text © 2009 Sonya Lennon and Brendan Courtney
Editing, design and layout © 2009 Merlin Publishing

Except
Photographs by Kip Carroll © Merlin Publishing/RTÉ
Photograph on page 179, © Lorna Fitzsimons

ISBN 978-1-907162-03-9

All rights reserved. No part of this book may be reproduced or utilised in any form or by any means electronic or mechanical, including photocopying, filming, recording, video recording, photography, or by any information storage and retrieval system, nor shall by way of trade or otherwise be lent, resold or otherwise circulated in any form of binding or cover other than that in which it is published without prior permission in writing from the publisher.

The publishers have made every reasonable effort to contact the copyright holders of photographs reproduced in this book. If any involuntary infringement of copyright has occurred, sincere apologies are offered and the owner of such copyright is requested to contact the publisher.

A CIP catalogue record for this book is available from the British Library.

10 9 8 7 6 5 4 3 2 1

Design: An Atelier project / www.atelier.ie
Printed and bound by Livonia Print, Latvia

OFF THE RAILS **LOVE YOUR LOOK**
TABLE OF CONTENTS

introduction
6 **WHY WE WANTED TO WRITE THIS BOOK**

chapter 1
10 **WHAT THIS BOOK CAN DO FOR YOU**

chapter 2
26 **IDENTIFYING YOUR BODY SHAPE**

chapter 3
46 **SEE THE BIG PICTURE**

chapter 4
60 **THE IMPORTANCE OF WEARING THE RIGHT SIZE BRA**

chapter 5
70 **EVERYTHING YOU ALWAYS WANTED
TO KNOW ABOUT SHAPEWEAR**

chapter 6
80 **NOW STYLE YOURSELF GORGEOUS**

chapter 7
124 **HOW TO ACHIEVE A FULLY FUNCTIONING WARDROBE**

chapter 8
136 **LEARN TO LOVE COLOUR**

chapter 9
146 **HOW TO SHOP**

chapter 10
166 **TIPS FROM THE EXPERTS**

180 SHOPPING GUIDE

191 CONCLUSION

ACKNOWLEDGEMENTS

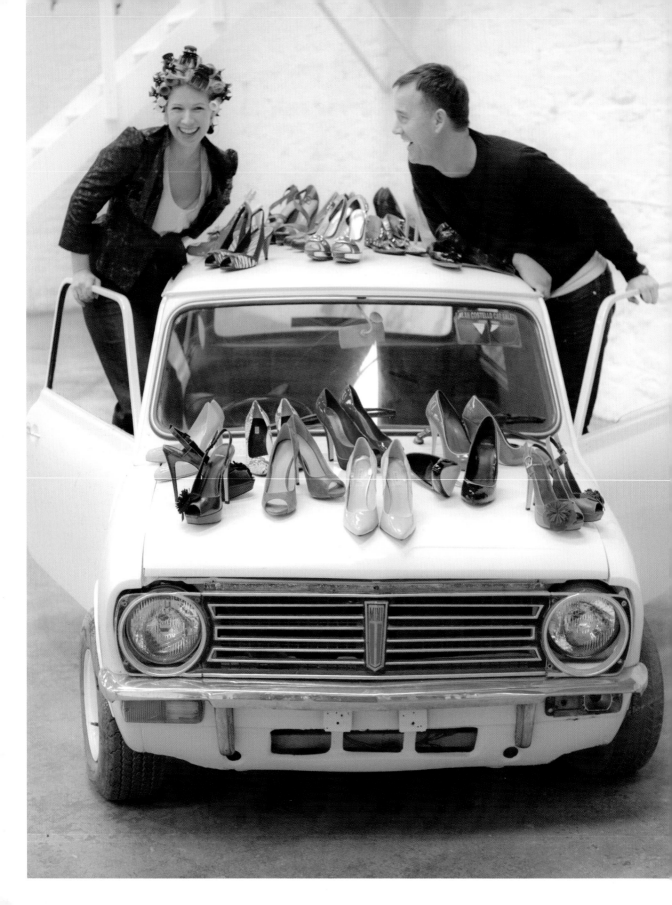

WHY WE WANTED TO WRITE THIS BOOK

We love our work, and we love working with each other. We also believe that our combined experience and understanding offer a comprehensive and uniquely Irish approach to the pursuit of looking good.

We are often approached by someone who is looking for advice, but does not want to go on the show. We enjoy talking to women about their different style queries, and as the number of queries has increased, we decided that the best way to get our message out there was to put pen to paper. So, to spread the gospel to a wider audience, this book was created.

We believe that whatever your body shape, you can look fantastic. It's incredible how infectious a positive attitude is. Our posture, body language and, by extension, the clothes we wear send signals to the world about how we would like to be perceived. A confident woman walks half a head taller than a woman who isn't happy with herself, whether she is 4ft 9" or 6ft 2". Our aim is that our readers will improve their self-confidence, as well as picking up some great style advice.

Many things can affect our self-confidence. It seems that no matter how gorgeous you are, most women have parts of their body they don't like. We fuel these thoughts with

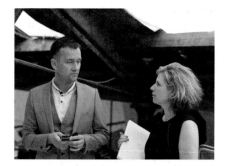

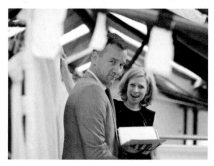

celebrity envy. Remember, you are women, not celebrities with nutritionists, trainers and endless time and resources to perfect your physiques.

To break this destructive cycle, something very fundamental needs to happen. We need to start loving ourselves as we are. It might sound too simplistic or silly, but it is the key to feeling great, whatever your shape or size. There is no perfect size to be in *real life*.

As well as a handbag, most modern women carry an 'If-list':

- If I could lose a stone
- If I could get to the gym twice a week
- If I could power-walk my way to a size 10

Some further accessorise with a 'Wish-list':

- I wish I were 2" taller
- I wish I had my sister's nose
- I wish I had skin like Beyoncé

These lists only add to our dissatisfaction and misery, and distract us from seeing our perfectly good bodies that can be draped to create a happy, stylish, sexy woman.

Anyone who has watched us in action will know that our philosophy for feeling good about our bodies is to focus on the positive. This is not the last time you will hear that piece of advice! When we begin to let kind feelings about ourselves into our lives, our confidence grows and our ability to change increases.

However, it's very difficult to begin the journey on your own. So we are here to guide you through the OFF THE RAILS experience, and teach you to love your look. The chances are, if you're reading this book, you have enjoyed watching the fabulous journeys of the amazing women that we transformed on the show. We started with tears of pain, and more often than not, ended with tears of joy. By reading this introduction, your journey has already begun.

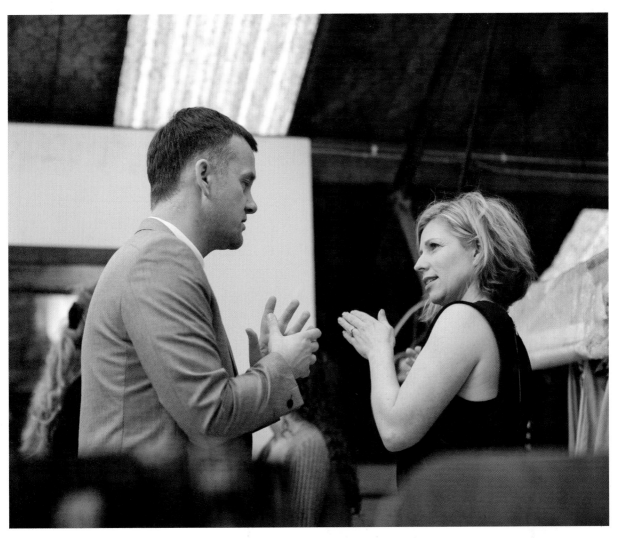

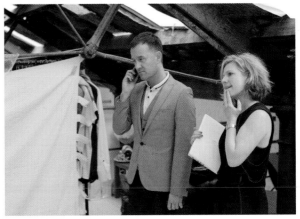

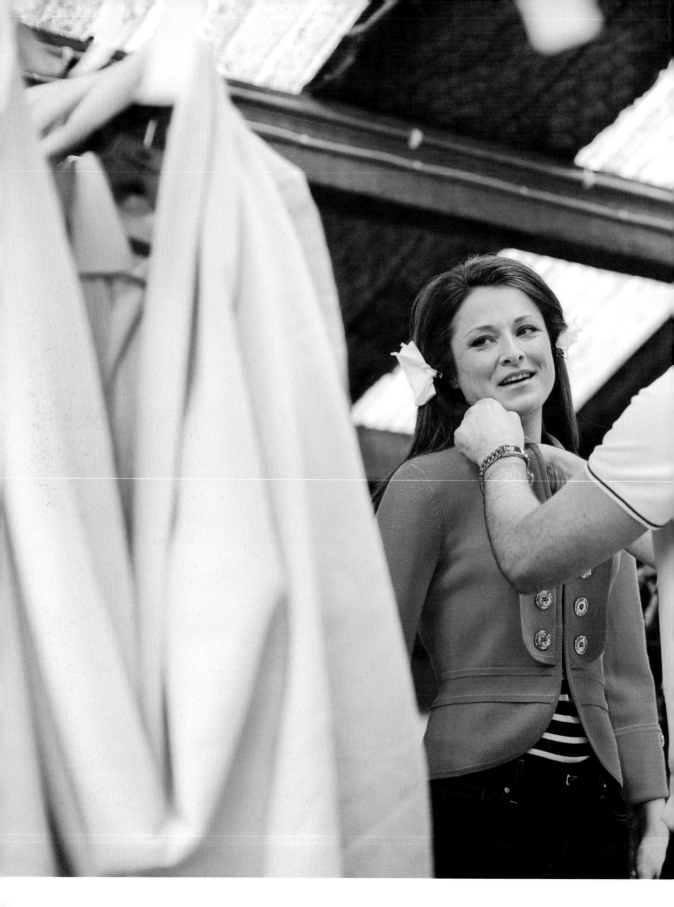

chapter one

1

WHAT THIS BOOK CAN DO FOR YOU

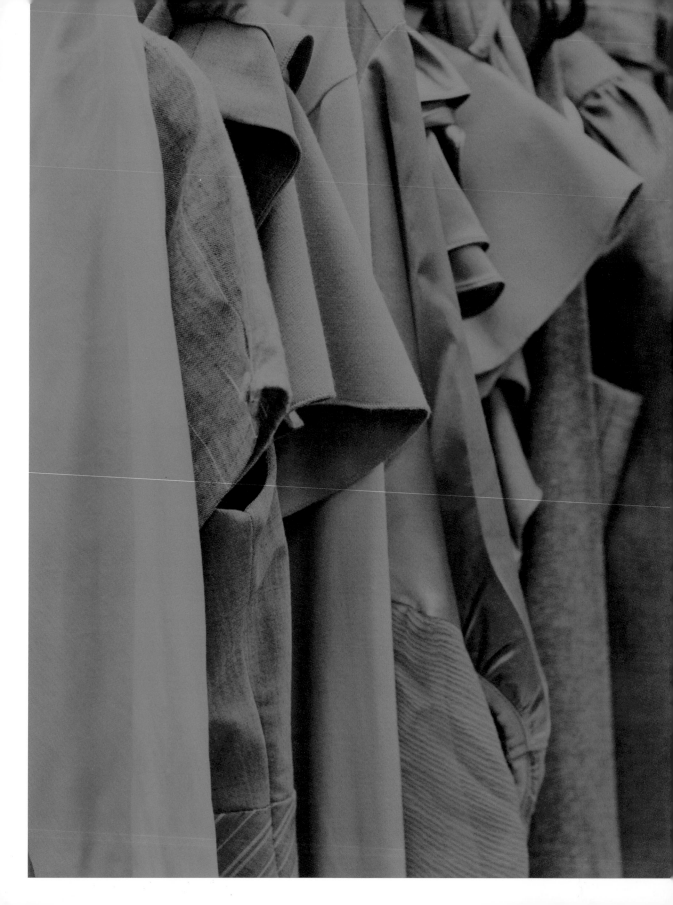

By writing this book we have attempted to give you your very own personal OFF THE RAILS experience. For instance, the wonderful transformations, growth of character, self-esteem building and, of course, the stunning styling that you see in the TV show are all yours for the taking. You will be able to have your very own 'make over' or, as we prefer to say, 'transformation', just by reading this book and applying our advice. You will look better and, therefore, feel a whole lot better about yourself.

The one thing that many of the women we have worked with have in common is lack of confidence and/or low self-esteem. For many of our girls on the show, this was not always the case, but life has a funny way of throwing some curveballs, and then all of a sudden our women found themselves unhappy with how they looked, and ultimately with who they were. So, the first thing we want this book to do for you, is to help you to start to like yourself more.

As a woman moves through the different stages of life: career, finding a partner, motherhood and beyond, she experiences different pressures and new anxieties, and often she stops considering herself. Frequently she ends up placing her happiness after everyone else's, and then the vicious circle happens, as her confidence and self-esteem spiral downwards.

The most tragic thing we ever heard was when a gorgeous women, in her late fifties, told us that not only could she remember the year but she could remember the exact hour that men stopped seeing her as an object of sexual desire! What is truly tragic about this statement is the number of women who can relate to it! The problem is one of perception, her perception of herself. In reality she can't see inside every

Leabharlanna Poibli Chathair Bhaile Átha Cliath
Dublin City Public Libraries

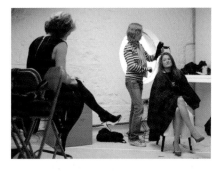

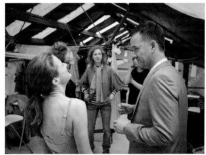

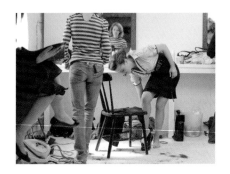

man's head and tell what he's thinking, so even on that level it cannot be true. But the awful truth is, if you feel like that woman did, you will make it your truth and it will affect you. So, we need to break the cycle, we need to show you that no matter what stage of your life you are at, it can be seen as a new chapter and a new opportunity to feel and look great.

We want to spread the message – how you look affects how you feel, and how you feel directly affects how you look, the two go hand in hand: if you look good you feel great, and when you feel great you look even better.

The very simple aim of our work is to make you see yourself positively.

We have learned that if a woman hates the way she looks, it is nearly always because she has gone through a period of not liking herself. What happens is, most people automatically focus on the things they don't like about themselves; fat bums, big thighs, or bingo wings. But this is such a waste of energy, and makes dressing oneself objectively impossible. It is really important that you pay attention to chapter 3, and pay particular attention to the part about loving your 'bits'. We are going to show you how to see only the best of yourself.

When you stop focusing on the bits of you that you don't like, and start to see, not only the good bits, but the whole picture (which, of course, is what everyone else sees), then you will start to feel better about yourself. At this point, finding the right clothes will no longer be a chore but a joy.

Every single woman we have worked with has shocked themselves by how much they changed and how exhilarating their experience was. And here's the good news; once this process occurred – with the right advice, they found it incredibly easy to see themselves in a new light.

Testimonials from our girls

'I learnt to explore and try new things on, even if they weren't something I would normally pick. It really was the best part for me.' **Samantha**

'It has had a huge effect on my life ... I now know how to dress to suit me and feel confident in what I'm wearing.' **Sonya**

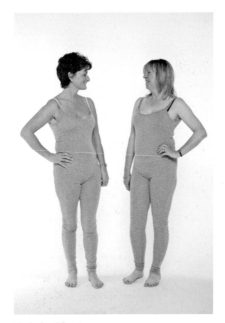

'Style buddies'

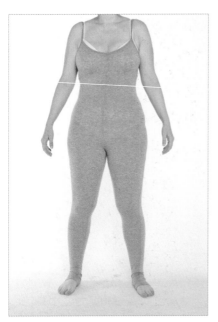

'The famous grey body suit'

Get a Style Buddy

So, here's an important observation: Irish women have great girl friends. Being Irish, we love to talk, and more often than not, it's our girl friends that we talk to. This is a natural resource that we are going to teach you to harness.

The first and only unpleasant aspect of all our on-screen transformations is the dreaded 'grey bodysuit'. So many of you have said that your enthusiasm for transformation has been tempered by the prospect of donning that dreadful garment. We don't like to linger on the bits of the body that cause anxiety, and neither should you. However, to really understand the potential of your body, you must be painfully honest with yourself. So, how about this, try using the theory of 'safety in numbers': choose a friend who you trust to help you out. You know who it is already – it's the girl who would bail you out of any situation. It's the girl who cocks her eyebrow to let you know that you may not have made the wisest decision. It's the woman who can do this while offering you a way out. So, use your girl friend, and let her use you as a beacon of honesty in the quest for style confidence.

What do you mean you don't have two hideous grey body suits lying around the house?

It's just the two of you, not 400,000 pairs of eyes. Strip down to your bra and knickers, and stand in front of the largest mirror you can find. Word of advice: find the mirror before you take off your clothes! Take turns to talk about what you see before you. Work methodically from your neck down to your toes. The important thing to do here is to be completely open and to really listen.

So, when you're at your most vulnerable, do the simplest thing. Get your style buddy to tighten your bra straps to the max, and if that doesn't make any difference, throw the bra in the bin.

After the honesty comes the resolution. Get your sweet feet out to a lingerie specialist, preferably one that carries a broad range of sizes. Don't go without your style buddy,

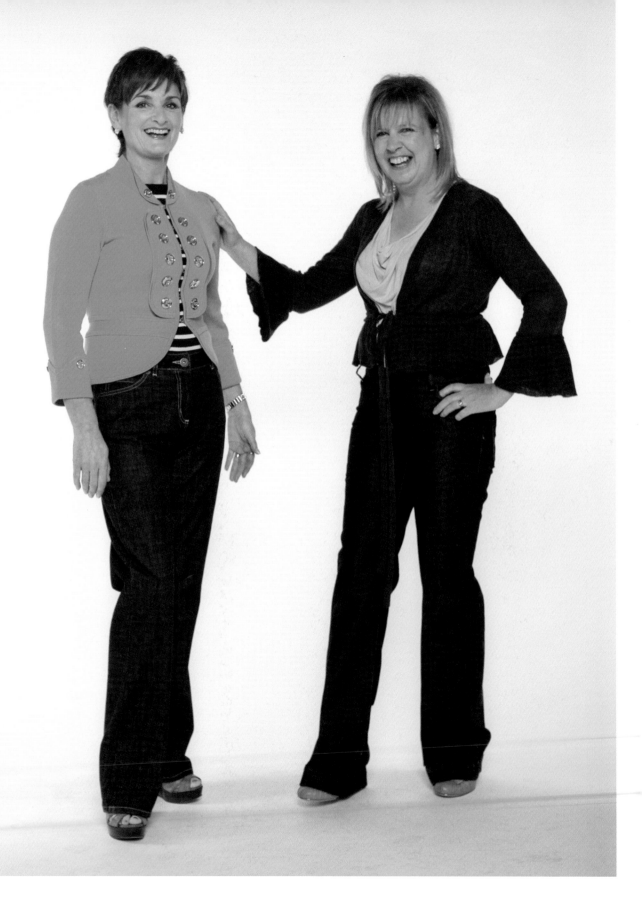

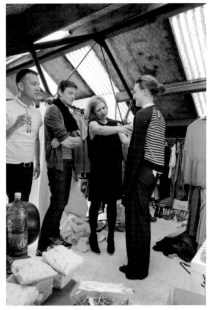

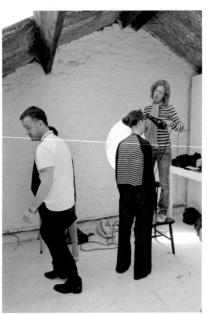

you're in this for the long haul now! Consider this trip like a visit to a medical professional, a non-surgical body lift, if you will. A good lingerie specialist can provide you with any number of solutions for your body issues. Magic underwear is the first step to wrangling your body and concealing the parts of it that are holding you back. Later in the book we will outline all you need to know about the mystical world of magic underwear, giving you the knowledge to make sure you get what you need for the task at hand.

So, now ladies you are fully loaded. Go back to the mirror and throw on a dress that would have brought you out in cold sweats, prior to enlightenment. You cannot fail to see that you are now taking control of your perceived failings. Suddenly you're at the driving wheel and in control.

The Dreaded S Word …

A unifying fact with all the women that we have helped is that they hate shopping. What? Hate shopping? But, all girls love shopping, right? Wrong. Shopping, unless you have the requisite knowledge, can be a scary prospect.

We have a full chapter in this book about how to tackle the assault course of the high street stores, chapter 8. From Topshop to Wallis, Brown Thomas to Dunnes Stores, it makes no difference; if you don't know what you're doing, clothes shopping can range from tricky to downright terrifying.

This is where your style buddy becomes invaluable. Together you can support each other through the process of rethinking your relationship with clothes, how to buy them and what they can do for you. So, how can your style buddy help you to shop? So many of you have told us that you find shopping intimidating and that you don't trust commission led, or worse, bored sales assistants.

Clothes shopping doesn't have to be a chore. This is supposed to be a woman's favourite pastime. So, what is the difference between style queens shopping with successful abandon from TKMaxx to high-end boutiques and the thousands of you that would rather sit at home than step into a changing room? The difference is confidence and knowledge.

Your style buddy and you act as a small army in the battlefield of the clothes shop. Remember that the customer is king (or queen). Once you believe that, you have no reason to be intimidated by snooty or ambivalent sales staff.

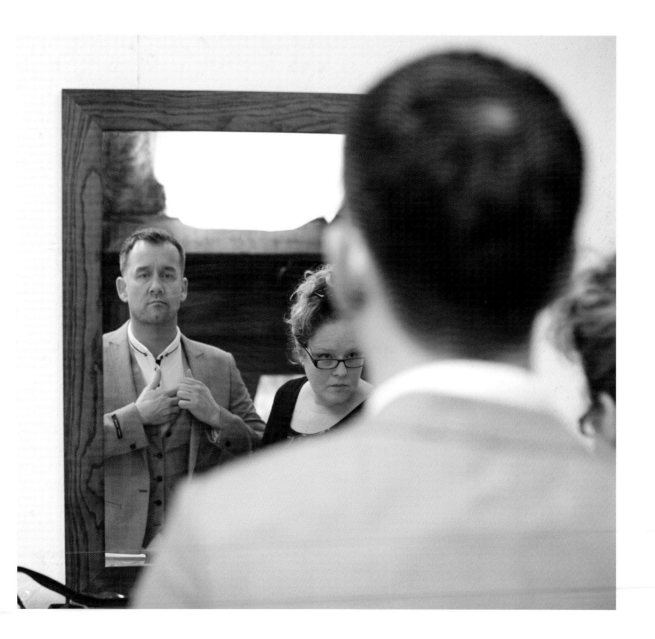

Work to a three-day plan and don't bring a credit card or any payment method with you until day three.

3-Day Programme

Day 1

Start with a calming cup of tea, and have a chat about what sort of things you would like to see on each other. Talk about colour and styles. Women often get stuck in a style rut.

This can be a reliance on anything from tracksuits to suiting. One has too little structure, and often the other has too much. The world of smart casual can be difficult to crack, follow chapter 6, to get the insider tips before you start.

Then go and try on with abandon! We guarantee you will laugh your socks off and even possibly end up in a pair of heels! Try on colours that you would never dream of, styles that you think are only for someone ten years your junior. If you hate patterns, go for the boldest ones you can find.

This is an exercise in bravery. Some pet hates you may lose, others may be rubber stamped, but try to have an open mind, and listen to your style buddy, that's why she's there.

Day 2

Again, start with a calming cup of tea. Talk about what worked on Day 1, and what really didn't. Now think about what you want out of your wardrobe. Any of the following?

- I want to look stylish in my casual clothes.
- I want to hold my head up high on the school run.
- I want to feel sexy and feminine in a work suit.
- I want a wardrobe full of clothes that work together.
- I want a wardrobe full of clothes I can wear.
- I want to ditch the black.

Think it through to avoid costly, pointless impulse buys. Or worse, endless re-buys of things that you already own. Now, hit the shops again – with a plan. Think about your best bits and accentuate them. What colours flatter your skin tone? Hold the colours right up to your face, don't be afraid! What items do you need? (See chapter 8)

Day 3

This is the big one! Get yourself a strong tea or coffee. Think back over Day 1 and Day 2.

- What did you try on that flatters your shape?
- What did you try on that really made you feel good?
- What did you try on that the 'new you' will wear?
- What did you try on that fits into your new colour palette. (See chapter 8)

Think about all the things that you tried on, that could live harmoniously together in your wardrobe and offer you more wardrobe choices than actual pieces. Now that is shopping clever.

When you have developed your grand plan, you have a framework from which to make future decisions. This does not mean that you can't break away from the plan. As confidence in your own ability grows, the potential to 'play' with clothes and have fun with your image also grows. Enjoy looking great!

Testimonials from our girls

'I notice things much more now, whereas before I didn't even really have the courage to say if I liked something or not ... I am much more confident now.' **Carol**

'I was never a fan of shopping, but I was very narrow-minded about clothes. I do enjoy it more now (if I had the money), and I buy completely different things than I used to.' **Aisling**

Guide to a successful transformation

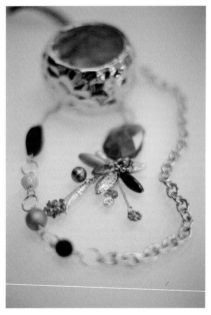

The road to a successful transformation in any area of your life can be, and often will be a challenging one. This does not mean that it is going to be terribly difficult, it just takes a little effort, application and commitment to achieve a successful outcome. All our ladies have said that the rewards far outweigh any bumps along their transformation journey. But the bright light at the end of the tunnel, the pot of gold at the end of the rainbow or, to put it simply, the rewards – are worth the effort. Just ask any one of the women we have worked with. With words like effort and commitment, it sounds like we are describing a marriage – well in a way we are! Think of this process as the beginning of the new relationship you have with yourself. It's now time to do a little work so that you can really learn to love yourself and how your look.

It's like anything that's worth doing, when you have completed it, you'll look back and realise that it was so much easier than you thought. We want this process to be so much fun that you will wonder why you didn't do it years ago. Think of it this way: the fact that you are reading this book is the start of your journey. Now, the most important part of your journey is – action. The ideas and exercises we show you throughout the book are the simplest way to becoming the new you.

These simple steps are the ingredients to your successful transformation.

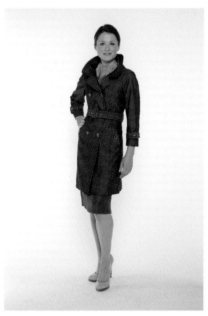

- A little effort (using a notebook to record any tips or guidelines along the way)
- Application
- Commitment
- Start loving yourself

The final result is the wonderful reward of gasping at your reflection in the mirror. Yes, that head-turner is you!

A LITTLE EFFORT

One of the few complaints that we got from our women was that they found it difficult to retain all the valuable information that we imparted. With that in mind, we encourage our ladies to keep a special notebook while they are going through the process. They record personal notes, ideas and any of our tips that grab their attention. This is also a great way to keep your mind focused on the task at hand. We like to think of our book as a manual that will last you for years. You might even like to paste a 'before' and 'after' photo of yourself in your notebook, as a reminder of your successful transformation.

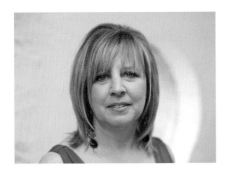

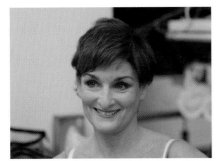

APPLICATION

We all have busy lives, that is why most of us, at some stage, get lost when it comes to style. What we suggest you do now is to factor your style transformation into your busy schedule. It might sound difficult, but you know the old saying, 'If you want something done, ask a busy person'. So, when you start to read this book, apply yourself as if you want to get full marks. Take the book as a unit, and travel trough it on your own personal journey from beginning to end, at your own pace, but at an applied pace. That way the benefits of the journey don't get broken by stopping and starting. We guess really what we are trying to do here is spur you on to be motivated to primarily enjoy this book, but also to get the best possible value from spending your precious time reading it.

COMMITMENT

Your relationship with yourself up until now may have been a little overlooked, maybe even a little neglected. Partner, friends, family, children and work, you've made a commitment to all of the above. We now urge you to make a commitment to yourself and this book. This means finishing the book, committing to the exercises and having fun trying them all out. As with all your relationships, when you commit to the process you give it your best shot.

START LOVING YOURSELF

Like any important relationship in your life, the relationship with yourself is just as valid and worth just as much effort

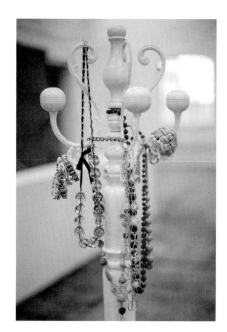

as all the others. Brace yourself for some 'personal development speak'. It is widely understood that: if you don't love yourself first, then it is difficult for others to love you and, therefore, meet your needs. Life shows you that you are ultimately responsible for your own happiness. In simple terms, you are so much easier to love, when you truly love yourself. This book will gently teach you how to start liking yourself, and hopefully, to start to truly love yourself, because, as far as we are concerned – you are fab!

Rewards

This is the best part of 'how to get the most out of this book', because when you do all of the above (even just a little), you will start to see the rewards immediately. And nothing keeps us going like a positive outcome, it's like when you lose that extra pound, or you save that €50, or you receive positive feedback from your boss – well this book works just like that, as it will motivate you to do more. We guarantee that you will see results and feel better the minute you start to apply our suggestions. One simple exercise, which we expand on in chapter 4, is something as simple as tightening your bra straps (wait until you see the effect of the magic knickers), by doing this you will immediately feel and see the benefits. You will not only enjoy seeing the benefits, but will also be motivated by them, and you will get the absolute maximum from this experience.

'Think about what you want to get out of it beforehand. Go in with a very open mind and a written list of every fashion/make-up question you ever wanted to ask.' **Máire**

'Be open minded and listen to the logic behind what you are told. You will never remember all the good advice; and the current fashion trends will go, but if you can understand where it's coming from you'll get a lot more out of the experience.' **Bernadette**

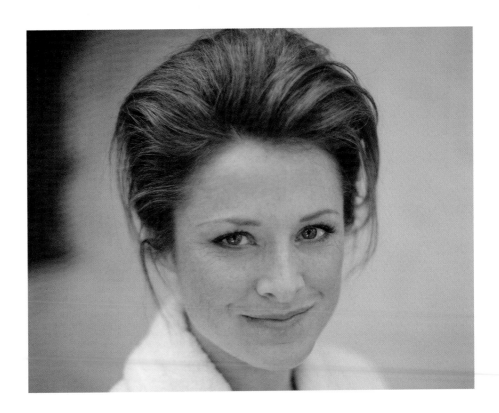

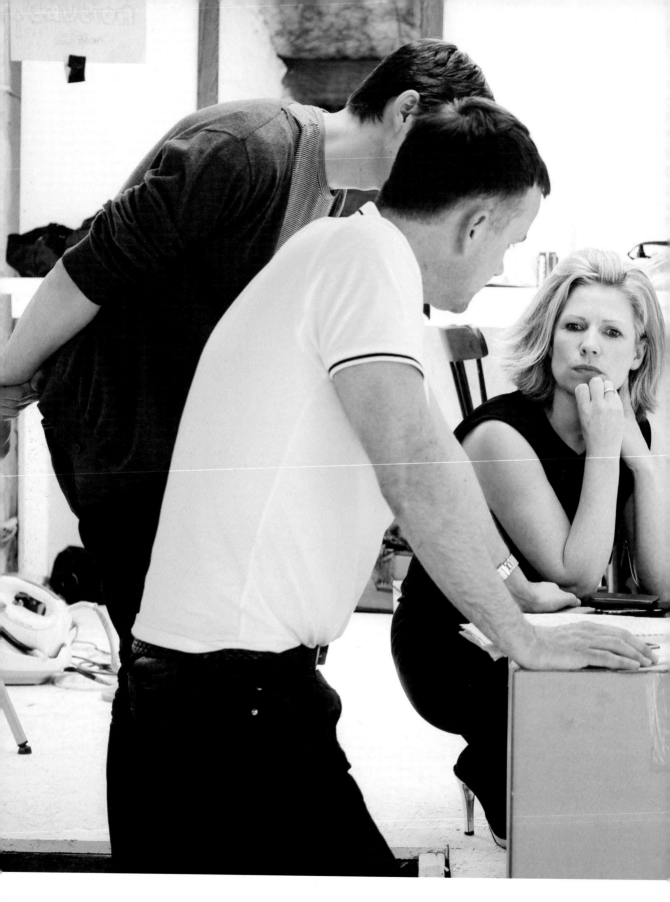

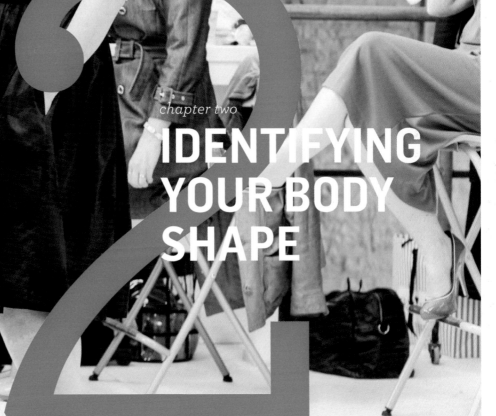

chapter two

2 IDENTIFYING YOUR BODY SHAPE

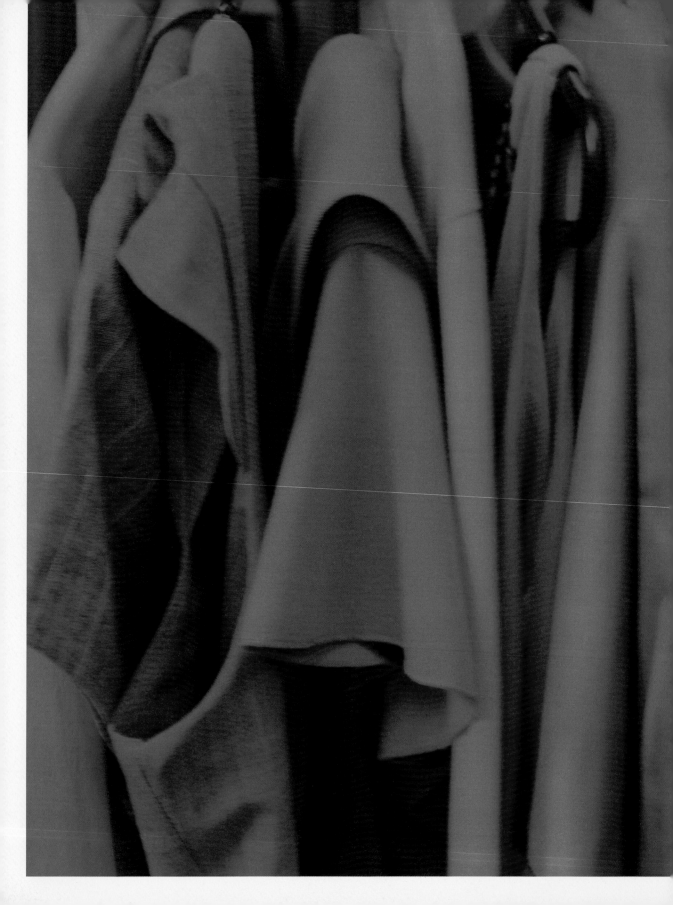

This is an essential exercise to do before you begin your transformation. By finding out which shape, or combination of shapes you are, you can begin to work towards achieving the super confident new you. Think of an awareness of your body shape as being the foundations of a majestic house. By evaluating your body shape you are also finding out the positive aspects of your shape, the ones you can emphasise and highlight. So, think of it as an exercise that will help you become aware of your best physical attributes. You may discover that your 'small' shoulders are perfect for fitted jackets, your 'full' hips look fantastic in a pencil skirt or your 'flat' chest is very elegant in a silk blouse.

Once you have identified your correct shape, you can use this as the basis for your transformation. To make things simple, we have selected the six most common body shapes: Pear, Apple, Ruler, Hour-glass, Petite and Amazonian. These are not the absolute gospel of body shapes, but merely a guide. Some women might identify with a combination of shapes, this is quite common. What we suggest here is that you take the elements from each body shape that apply to you and combine them. This is creating a solid foundation from which to build the new magnificent you.

The grey body suit

Not only is pinpointing your body shape a fundamental and important part of the OFF THE RAILS process, but can also be really fun. Some might say it appears to be the most painful and embarrassing part of our TV transformations, especially the part where we put our gorgeous gals in a skin-tight grey body suit. (Incidentally we don't get our ladies down to their knickers, because we believe this process is actually about making them feel good, not humiliating them, and we believe the grey suit protects their modesty, so our gals can stand there with a modicum of dignity!)

The super important job that this allows us to do is:

- evaluate the body shape
- demonstrate the importance of wearing the correct size bra
- show the incredible power of magic support underwear (more about these later in chapter 5, now back to basics!).

All our girls will testify that once you 'just do it' or 'take the plunge', the body analysis is actually not too bad, and the benefits far outweigh the embarrassment. The really clever bit is that you get to do it in the privacy of your own home and not with the entire nation watching you on RTÉ One!

Think of it this way – if we didn't start with the body analysis we couldn't do our job. Apart from the importance of knowing the body shape and proportions for styling, it is useful to demonstrate how wearing the correct size bra affects the body shape and wearing the right shapewear can boost body confidence. This is also the time when we get to look at what it is our girls hate about their bodies – so if it's their bums or their thighs or their arms, we can start to re-train their eye to see themselves as a whole unit, thus gaining perspective on their own shape. This is also where we introduce them to the good stuff they don't see; lovely boobs, great waist, long legs or whatever those overlooked assets might be.

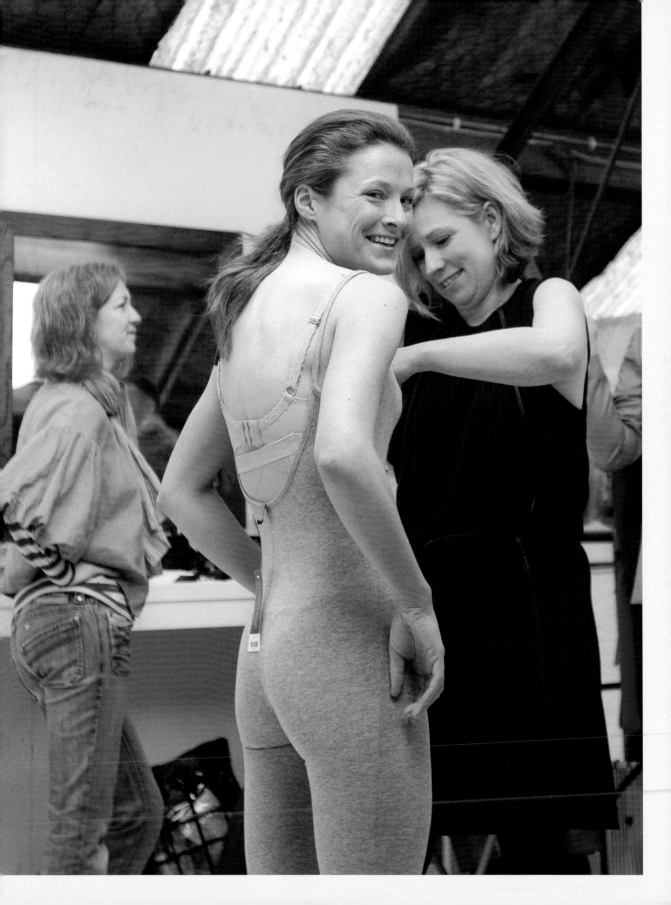

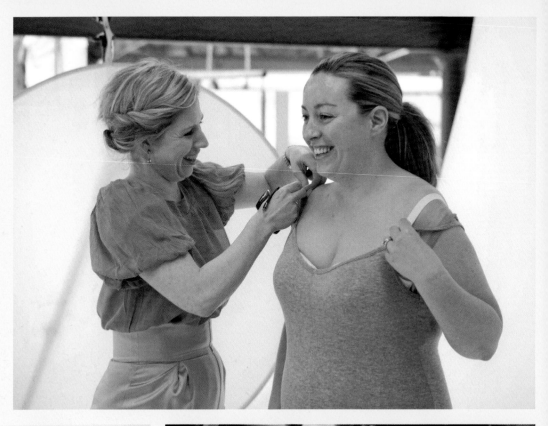

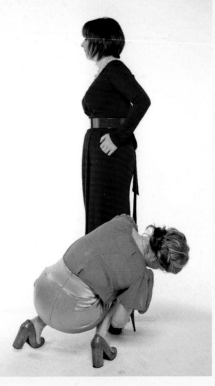

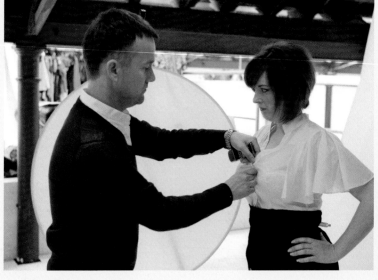

◄ *It's not all glamorous!*

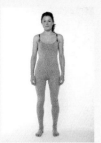

Petite

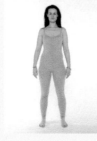

Amazonian

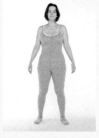

Apple

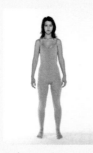

Pear

Hour-glass

Ruler

It is essential to remember that everybody has attractive aspects that they are often unaware of. This point applies to you as well, so take note! This process is incredible, because most of the time our women are amazed at how many good features they possess that years of negative body image and thinking has made them blind to. It's wonderful for us to then witness, once the positive aspects have sunk in, the growth in their confidence and their ability to start to feel good about themselves.

But the really, really important part of this process for you is very simple and very valuable – it's just about getting you back in front of the mirror. We promise you the more time you spend in front of the mirror looking at the bits you like – the better you will feel, because you will become re-familiarised with yourself. It is like the first time you see yourself on video, you are always surprised at how you sound and how you look; well this process is about getting to know yourself and the more time you spend at it and work at seeing the positive, the more you will like yourself and the better you will feel and, ultimately, the better you will look.

(We also advise at this point that you get your style buddy on board.) Get down to your bra and knickers, and analyse each other. Remember, it's great to have another set of eyes to be objective. It's also good to have someone to compare your shape and size to. If however, this notion is just too embarrassing for you, you can use the six images of our gorgeous ladies to help you diagnose your body shape. Our lovely models have agreed to act as a guide for you, as they have been through the process and are aware that it might be initially uncomfortable, but highly beneficial. Just decide who you are closest to in body shape, remember this is not an exact science and there are no rules – no right and wrong – rules are for school! These photographs act as a guide. You can even take someone's top half and combine it with another of our women's lower body, in order to get the best results for you.

PEAR

Upper body
You usually have a neat torso
with narrow shoulders.

Mid-section
You tend to have a small waist.

Lower body
Your lower half is larger than
your top half (and remember,
its never as big as you think).

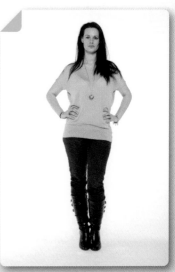

Nadia before her transformation

PEAR

BEYONCÉ, SHARON OSBOURNE, KATHRYN THOMAS, SHAKIRA
and KRISTIN DAVIS (CHARLOTTE FROM SEX AND THE CITY)

Young mum of two, Nadia Power comes from Rush, and is married to Jason. She finds her Pear shape frustrating to style. Nadia, have no fear – this über womanly silhouette is a joy to dress; just apply a few simple rules! Nadia finds it difficult to get the correct size bra for her post-baby body, and at 5ft 8", she would love to find the right length jeans.

Great news Pear shapes – you are the most common shape of all. It is important to note that Pear shapes are not all the same, as you can see from our celebrity list above. You are as diverse as the skinny Pear, Kristin Davis, and the more rounded and mature Pear, Sharon Osbourne. There is not a single size for a single Pear – you come in all sizes.

How do you figure out if you are a delicious Pear? With typical Pear shapes, your lower half is larger than your top half (and remember, it's never as big as you think!). For the record, statistics reveal that men are most attracted to this womanly shape.

You tend to have a small waist, which can be made look even smaller by your larger hips. And, typically, most Pears have a neat torso with narrow shoulders. The brilliant thing about your delicate little waists, is that it makes our job a pure pleasure. But we need to get your eyes off those hips, thighs and bum, and focus on your slender top half. You tend to focus on your bum, thighs and saddlebags, instead of looking up at your torso and at your glorious waist. You have a relatively flat stomach and great arms. Often Pear shapes have wonderfully pert breasts. Fashion has started to celebrate your shape, with the re-emergence of '40s fashion.

Tip Celebrate your tiny waist and neat torso. Rejoice in your womanly curves and your bootilicious bum. You have a very easy silhouette to dress, and a super fun shape to make look sexy.

APPLE

Upper body
The classic Apple has a wide back and a large chest and lovely arms

Mid-section
You tend to have a rounded tummy.

Lower body
You have enviable slender legs.

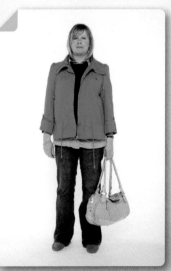

Teresa before her transformation

APPLE

BETH DITTO, DREW BARRYMORE, KATE WINSLET
and BLÁTHNAID NÍ CHOFAIGH

Our delicious Apple, Teresa Kelly is 40-something and she has five sons. Needless to say, she has her hands full. Teresa hates shopping, and finds it really difficult to buy clothes that flatter her figure.

Some of the most confident sexy women are Apple shaped. Beth Ditto not only celebrates her shape, but inspires all Apples to push the boundaries. She has shown that with confidence you can look beautiful and sexy, no matter what your shape or size. At first glance, you might be forgiven for thinking Apple shapes are not well catered for on the high street, but with some of our very simple tricks and advice, we can help you look and feel a million dollars.

How do you know if you are a delicious Apple? You have slender legs and lovely arms. Apples tend to have a wider back and a large chest with a rounded tummy. Often, you think your biggest problem is that your tummy is larger than your breasts. Don't fret, this is not a problem. A lot of other shapes envy your slim legs, flat bum and ample bosom.

Your extremities are your best feature, and as we've said, we need to get those boobs and that belly into the best possible support underwear (scaffolding). For your shape, it is so important to wear the right bra, because how good you look is dictated by where your boobs are. And don't despair, if you think you don't have a waist, we will show you how to find it. In our experience, Apple shapes tend to have the lowest confidence of all the shapes. It may at first appear tricky to dress you, but let us assure you it is NOT. You have the best arms and legs of all the shapes. You also have boobs to die for – you just haven't been showing them off!

You tend to obsess about your tummy. You feel it overshadows everything else. Wearing larger clothes makes you look ten times larger than you actually are. You are a woman, and we need to celebrate that with what your wear.

 Tip You often don't see your fabulous legs or lovely slender arms; you can be completely unaware of your gorgeous décolletage (the area between your neck and chest!).

RULER

Upper body
Rulers often have long torsos.

Mid-section
Your hips and shoulders tend to be the same width as your waist.

Lower body
For your height, you may have short legs.

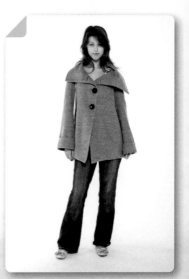

Alison before her transformation

RULER

NICOLE KIDMAN, TILDA SWINTON, JEAN BUTLER, JOANNA LUMLEY and YVONNE KEATING

Twenty-two year old Alison O'Riordan from Tullamore is a student at DCU, studying international business and languages. At 5ft 8" Alison has real trouble getting clothes to fit, and give her the curves she wants.

Rulers, you are the most unusual of our shapes. You get the least amount of sympathy from other women, because you are tall, slender and sleek! Other shapes can't see what your problem is, but often Rulers can have disproportion between their torsos and their legs, and can actually find it very difficult to find suitable clothes.

Our list of celebrity Rulers reads like a who's who of the world's most beautiful women, so it is easy to see why other women have little or no sympathy for our ravishing Rulers. Probably the most famous Ruler, Nicole Kidman highlights her proportions perfectly. With a long torso, she rarely exposes her legs above the knee. Joanna Lumley always looks chic and perfectly proportioned.

Your hips and shoulders tend to be the same width as your waist, which is often not as defined as you would like. Some Rulers feel that their legs are disproportionately shorter than their torsos. What most people don't know is that many Rulers can have large thighs in comparison to their general slenderness. What you don't tend to see is that to the rest of the world you look like a supermodel.

We can show you how to get the best from your gorgeous shape and re-structure your proportions to diva dimensions! Using volume and proportion, we will show you how to maximise your model-like silhouette.

 Tip Elegant Ruler, your ideal skirt length is below the knee.

HOUR-GLASS

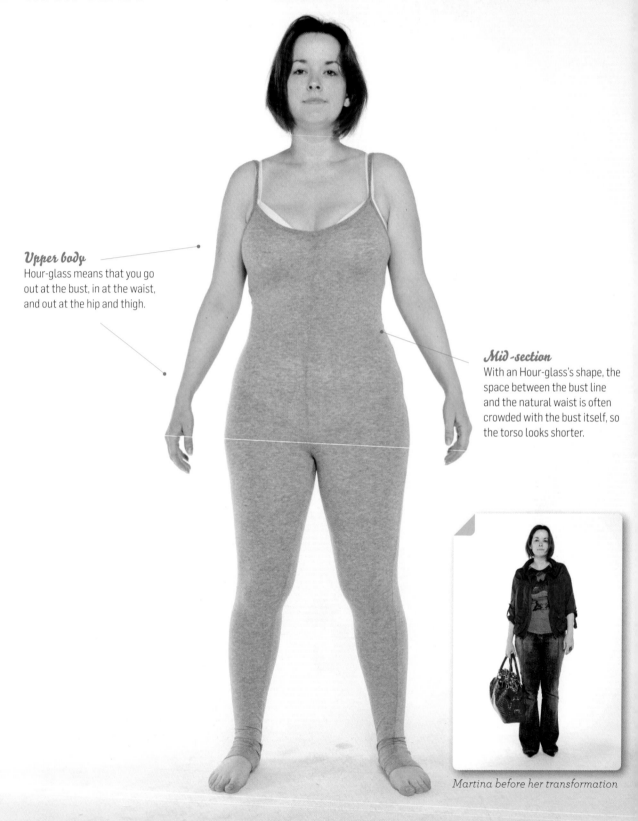

Upper body

Hour-glass means that you go out at the bust, in at the waist, and out at the hip and thigh.

Mid-section

With an Hour-glass's shape, the space between the bust line and the natural waist is often crowded with the bust itself, so the torso looks shorter.

Martina before her transformation

HOUR-GLASS

MARILYN MONROE, HELEN MIRREN, SCARLETT JOHANSEN, GRÁINNE SEOIGE and AMANDA BRUNKER

Thirty-three year old Martina Dignam is our fabulous Hour-glass, and has lost a whopping three stone and three lbs in the past few months. With her new found confidence, Martina finds shopping a joy, but sometimes doesn't know how to dress her new shape.

How do you know if your are an Hour-glass shape? Very simply, Hour-glass means that you go out at the bust, in at the waist and out again at the hip and thigh. No matter what your dress size is, the important element to get right is proportion. A large bust is a powerful asset, if used correctly. The very first thing you have to do is check that bra size. This is the beginning of changing your relationship with your shape, so invest wisely in the foundations. If you try to camouflage your shape with baggy clothes – we promise you that you will look ten times bigger.

Very often, a woman's narrowest point is her back, just below the bust. With an Hour-glass shape the space between the bust line and the natural waist is often crowded with the bust itself, so the torso looks shorter. Definition of the waist area is the key to success. Even if you think your waist should be narrower, it's still the punctuation for what lies above and beneath it. Lift that bust high. Most women are wearing their bra straps too long, so lift them high to lengthen the torso area.

What you've got is a classic sexy body shape, so think about how the icons listed maximise their assets. Don't be tempted to go half way with that favourite garment of the body shy – the empire-line. You need to follow the contours of your body right down to your natural waist, and beyond!

So, you think your hips are too big! Women are supposed to have hips, that's why people often refer to your shape as 'womanly'. The trick is to bring the eye out at the curves and then in again. The pencil skirt is the perfect garment to help you celebrate what you have. Just make sure that it's fitted to the knee, not hanging straight down from the hip.

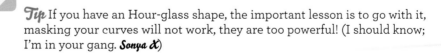

Tip If you have an Hour-glass shape, the important lesson is to go with it, masking your curves will not work, they are too powerful! (I should know; I'm in your gang. *Sonya X*)

PETITE

Upper Body

Anyone 5ft 4" or under can be comfortably described as Petite.

Lower body

Often Petites have small feet and it can be difficult to find shoes that fit.

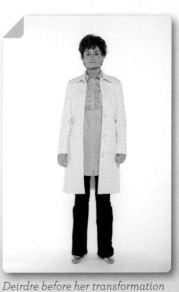

Deirdre before her transformation

PETITE

KYLIE, MADONNA, EVA LONGORIA, LULU and ANDREA CORR

Deirdre O'Neill is a 44 year old home maker from West Dublin. She is also Teresa's (our Apple) best friend and neighbour. Deirdre is married with two kids, Donna and Karl. She says she is incredibly indecisive, and as a result often comes home empty handed from a shopping trip. Deirdre has short legs and is self-conscious about her belly (We know! What belly?).

Anyone 5ft 4" or under can be comfortably described as Petite. Petite is only a reference to your height, and you can be Petite and any combination of the other body shapes, with the obvious exception of Amazonian.

Being small brings with it very specific issues. Quite often, Petites have small feet and it can be difficult to find shoes to fit. There are a limited number of stores that carry smaller sizes, but our advice is to get to work at the keyboard. See our shopping guide for the best place to purchase smaller than average size shoes.

If your body is in this category then your potential to look breath-taking is huge. However, without a celebrity's army of stylists it can be difficult to find clothes in this size, as the smallest standard high street size is 8 (Topshop and Miss Selfridge carry size 6). Again, our advice is to use the internet. It's not a shopping substitute, but it can provide solutions. See our shopping guide for listings.

If your body does not contain itself to these tiny proportions, all is not lost. A few key guidelines can help you to give the impression that you are taller than you are.

Follow the contours of your body with your clothes. Any flowing camouflage on a smaller frame will just push you down even more. Try to dress in one solid colour head to toe or in varying shades of the same tone, as this lengthens what the eye sees. Follow our guidelines in chapter 6.

 Tip Try heels, they are the simplest and most effective way to make you look taller. As well as heels, the wedge and the platform are the little gal's best friend. Avoid ankle straps though, as they shorten the look of the leg.

AMAZONIAN

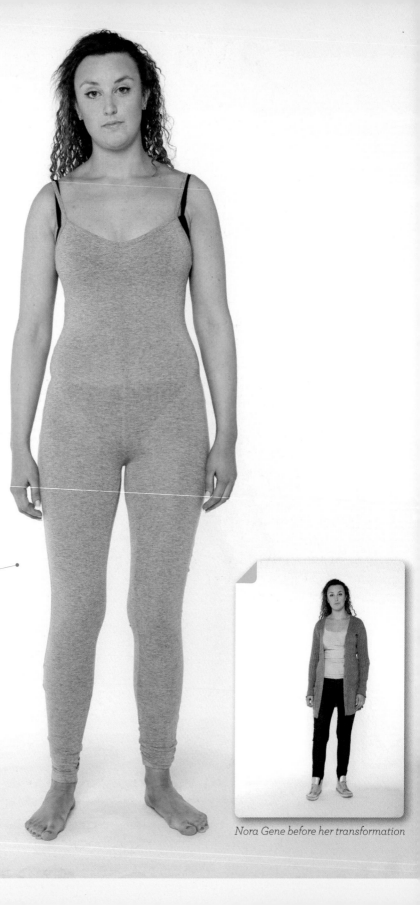

Upper body
Good posture is essential for the taller girl.

Lower body
You have enviable long legs.

Nora Gene before her transformation

AMAZONIAN

ELLE MCPHEARSON, BROOKE SHIELDS, UMA THURMAN and
MIRIAM O'CALLAGHAN

Nora Gene O'Connor is a 25 year old Limerick lass. At 5ft 9" she finds length a real issue. She would kill for a good tailored jacket that actually fits. Nora Gene works in press and promotions, so looking smart is very important. Also, finding the right trousers would be a blessing for her!

You lucky lady! It's safe to say that if you are 5ft 9", or over, and in proportion to your height, you are a warrior queen! We've helped some incredibly tall women during the series, specifically because many of them aren't comfortable with their gift of height. This is due to a couple of factors. They felt that they physically took up too much space and, also, they found it very hard to feel feminine.

There is nothing that we can do about our height, so the key is to celebrate it. Who says you can't be tall and feminine? It's not for nothing that catwalk models are generally 5ft 9" plus. The greater the height of the model – the more flow and drama for the outfit.

However, practical issues abound. A woman of 5ft 11" would look perfectly in proportion in a dress size 16–18, and in this crazy mixed up world, that is teetering at the edge of the world of 'Outsize'. Whoever called it that in the first place should face some serious retribution. Check out our shopping guide for insider tips on dressing your fabulous Amazonian frame.

If you are 5ft 10" or over with model proportions, for instance, size 8–10, you are probably more Svelte than Amazonian. Anyone identifying themselves in this category will get little sympathy from their less perfectly proportioned friends. However, if your height is a problem for you, then it's a problem. But that's why we wrote this book. Follow our tips in chapter 6, to learn how to see the glory in what you've got.

Tip Let us show you how to feel feminine without feeling silly and frilly. Think sexy rather than girly; it can be as simple as wearing a well-cut dress with a pair of pumps.

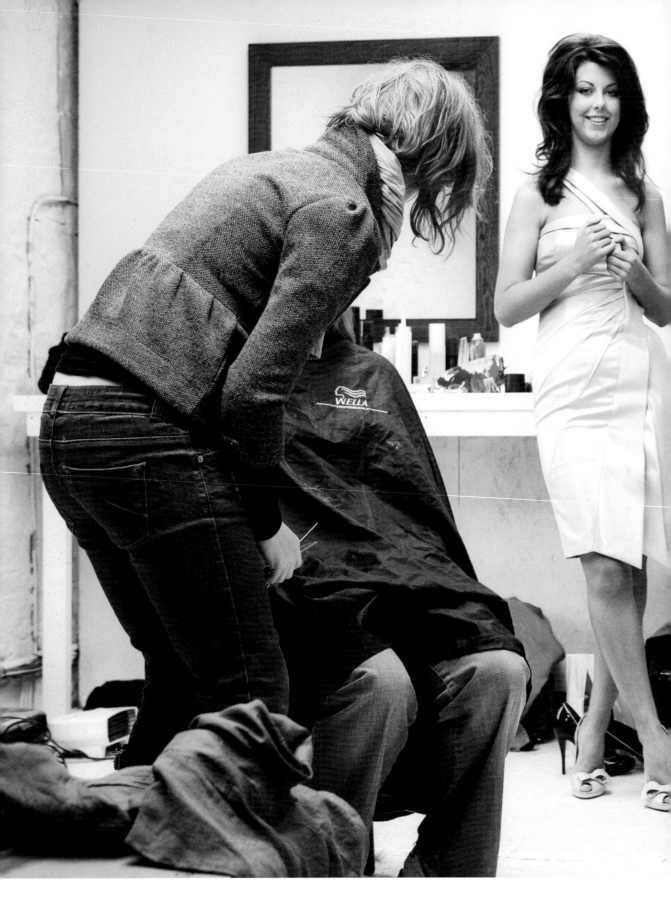

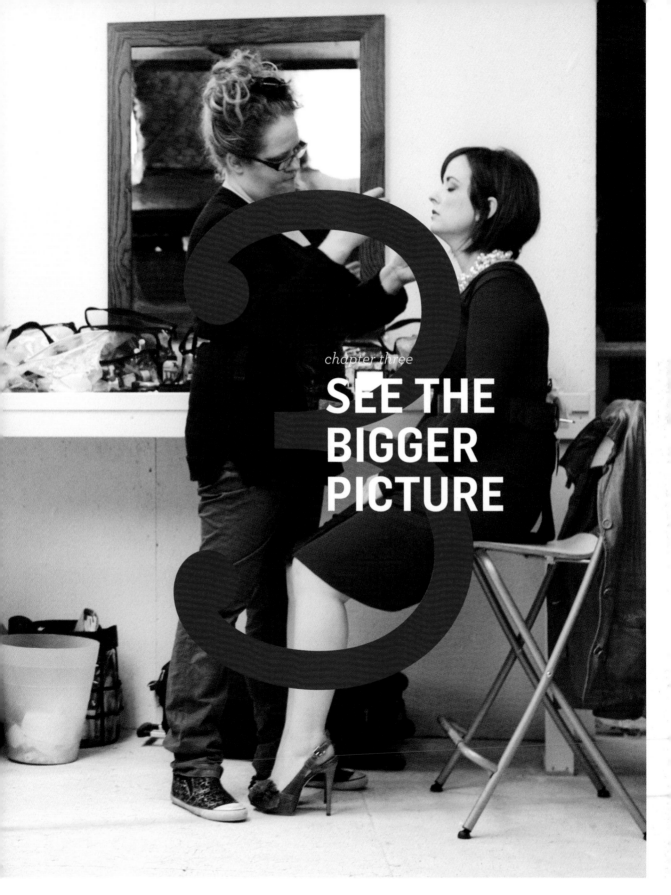

chapter three

SEE THE BIGGER PICTURE

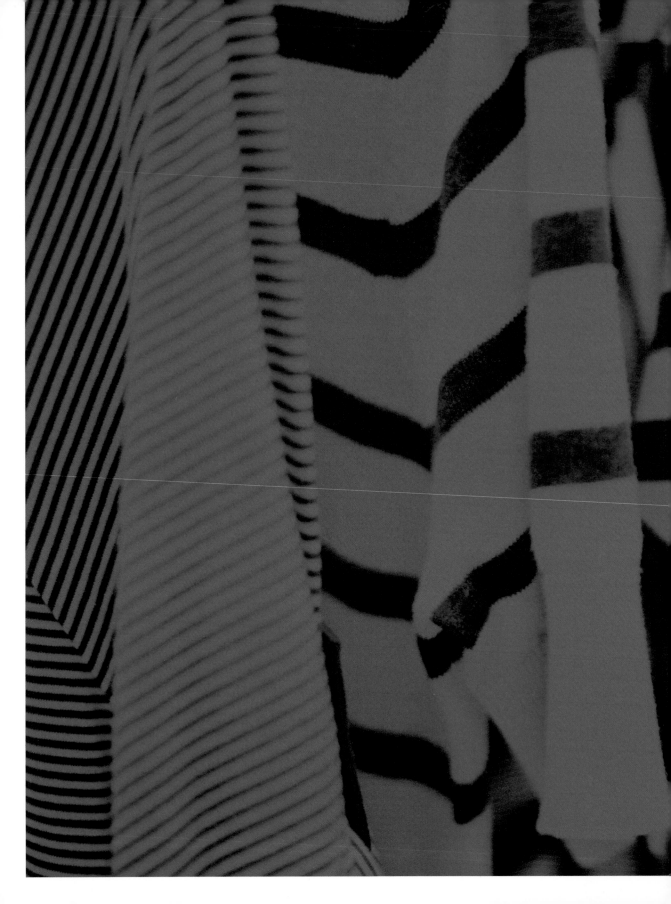

Identify what you don't like

Identifying the parts of your body that you don't like probably comes easily to most of you. However, emotionally it can be the trickiest part of the process, because practically everybody in the world can write an enormous list of what they hate about themselves physically (in most cases as long as your arm!). Invariably people will imagine things to be a lot worse than they actually are; to be objective about your own body is very difficult. This distorted view occurs for four reasons – learned thinking, vicious circle, pattern of negative thinking and unrealistic goals.

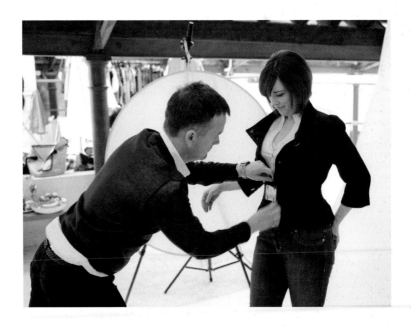

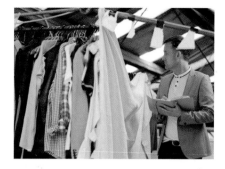

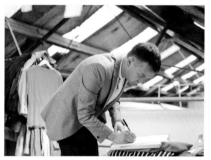

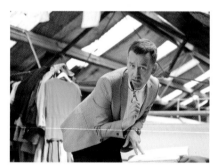

Learned thinking

As we get older we get stuck in our learned way of thinking – what we learned as children from our parents/guardians and teachers. We pick up their habits, and by the time we are adults this style of thinking is outdated. For example, traditionally, typical Irish thinking was to cover up our bodies, accompanied by feelings of guilt, and for the ordinary classes, a feeling that we 'weren't deserving or good enough'. In particular women, up to not so long ago, were considered second-class citizens. But girls we've come a long way! There are millions of historical reasons why we thought like this, but the scars of that thinking mean we often only see the negative. If we focus on the negative for long enough it becomes our reality. Thankfully, the older generation of women most affected by this thinking have now found their voice and (for the most part!) equal rights.

Vicious circle

By only seeing the negative, we don't see any positive. In life's worst vicious circle – the less positive we see the more negative takes over and it spirals downwards. The two go hand in hand. Positive thinking needs to happen to stop the negative, or else a pattern will occur!

Pattern of negative thinking

So, in summary, what we see in the mirror after years of negative thinking can be distorted. We need to look at ourselves in a positive light in order to break the pattern of negative thinking. The good news is that this cycle is easy to break, and we can show you how to liberate yourself of your negative body image. Ladies, it's time to move on.

Unrealistic goals

Coupled with all the demons in our heads, we also have to deal with the unrealistic goals portrayed in the media. Skinny models thrust radiant smiles and airbrushed limbs at us from the covers of magazines, TV and the internet daily. Movie star moms slip back into size 0 jeans with apparent ease, and juggle stellar careers with picture-postcard family life. This is not reality. We don't get to see the legions of hairdressers, make-up artists, nutritionists, personal trainers, stylists – and crucially – cosmetic surgeons, who all play their part in the multimillion dollar (and euro!) industry supporting the myth of perfection. All of this, coupled with our backgrounds and our desire for immediate results means further assaults on our self-esteem, and ultimately we set unrealistic goals. The notion of crash diets, starvation and endless workouts at the gym seem like mountains that cannot be climbed, particularly when our self-esteem is too low to sustain the ordeal.

Take our advice Learn to love yourself as you are first. When you achieve that, super human power is yours! Many of our transformation candidates have gone on to lose weight, and positively change their lifestyles simply because, for the first time in years, they felt they deserved it.

The body parts we hate and how to love them

By identifying clearly what it is that really bothers you about your body, we can work at breaking down your negative image of that area. Then we find the areas of the body you do like, and 'voila' show you how to get the most out of your entire body! This is where we start to gently introduce DEBS, which is:

D for distract or disguise our problem areas
E for emphasise the good parts or the bits you do like and feel work for you
B for balance. Keeping your body as an entire unit, using shape, detailing and colour to create balance
S for sexy, stylish and stunning, which is exactly how you will feel when you apply our ideas

A closer look at the most common pet 'body part' hates:

BUMS

Most Irish women's 'big issue' is their bums! Thus, most of our nation's curves get shrouded in big, baggy and unflattering clothes. But before we continue, it is the curve of your bum that creates one of the most impactful areas of your feminine silhouette, and the more this curves the more feminine it looks. So big is good, and not that it's important, but just nice to know that most men love a large bum and prefer it to a small one. Still not convinced? Well, dressing your bum to balance your proportion is easy, and there are loads of simple and clever ways to help you feel more comfortable and look gorgeous. We will show you how to do this in chapter 6. But remember Jay-Lo is better known for her gorgeous big bum then anything else, and she doesn't hide it under layers and anoraks.

Quick Fix Draw the eye up by adding detail to your top half; create balance with volume on the shoulder and in the sleeves. Try on a pencil skirt, this notion might send you reeling in horror, but you will be amazed at how Jessica Rabbit you can look, because a tight fit with a strong supported fabric will actually make you look sleeker!

THIGHS

Staying with the lower half, bums and thighs tend to go hand in hand in the hate stakes. Normally, most women who have a problem in this area have a problem with their entire lower half, and try to cover it up with baggy or ill-fitting clothes, never venturing into good jeans or trousers. Women who don't like their thighs can become obsessed with this area and blind to the beauty of the rest of their bodies. Using the same principles of distraction, we can get that area totally under control, and have you feeling fabulous.

Quick Fix Create balance with shoulder pads or voluminous sleeves. Highlight your waist with a good belt to make you appear more hour-glass. Most importantly, all lower garments (skirts, trousers, etc.) need to skim your hips, this way it disguises them and makes your legs look like they go on forever.

Apple shapes and women with post-baby tums tend to have the same hang-up – they hate their mid section. Even if your tummy is larger than your chest, don't panic, it is really not a problem. This is the problem area that can make any women go straight for black and baggy, adding to her discomfort about her appearance. Focusing on this area can be very distressing, as you feel everyone is looking at your belly. Well they are not, and it's only you who is aware of it and upset by it. With the right bra, and by making 'empire line' your new best friend, we can vastly improve how you feel about yourself and your yummy tummy (and that's just the tip of the iceberg, more on that later). There are lots of clever uses of shape and colour blocking, which will redefine your silhouette. And remember, it's never as bad as you think.

Quick Fix Lift those boobs with the right size bra, I know we are repeating this, but with tummy issues this really helps alleviate the problem. Empire line is your new best friend, that is any top or dress that has the waistband sitting just under your boobs (i.e. your narrowest point). A really good fitted jacket will completely redefine your torso, giving you a waist and slicing your silhouette to make you appear taller and sleeker. If you have tummy issues – remember to get those lovely legs and arms out.

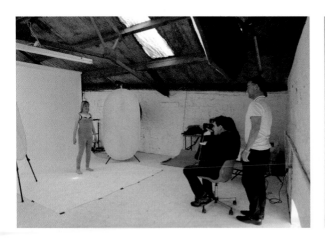
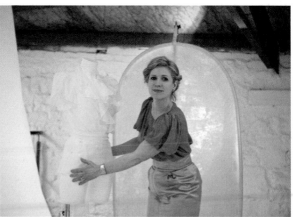

ARMS

We need to start a support group and call it, 'Women and Arms', as so many of you hate your arms. This area is easiest to tackle. We are constantly shown images of stick-thin models and actresses with long scrawny arms, and told this is how women's arms should look – this simply is not the case. Every time we have worked with a woman with an arm issue, we have resolved it in minutes. There are plenty of steadfast tricks of the trade for dealing with arm issues, which we guarantee will have you feeling much better about yourself.

Quick Fix Caped sleeves are genius for disguising but not swamping. Our 'fav' tip for this area is make the tailor your best friend. Buy a jacket one size up so your arms are comfortable and not squeezed into the sleeves, and then have the tailor adjust the jacket to fit you perfectly. Use your style buddy to objectively assess the area. Other tips: volume sleeves, kimono sleeves, puff shoulders and deep V-necks for distraction.

BOOBS

Too big or too small there is a bra for you, it's just about finding it and it's really not too difficult. But your boobs are your ultimate statement of femininity, and should never be hidden away – whatever size. Your boobs should make you feel womanly, and in styling terms, they are God's gift to reshaping any body type – you just need to be a little brave and not afraid to show a little cleavage from time to time. The three lessons we have learned when it comes to dealing with boobs are: support, support, support! You need to get the right size bra!

Quick Fix Stop what you are doing right now and tighten your bra straps! Hey presto, instant boob lift!

LEGS

Too short, too long or too wide, chunky calves, kankles (half calf half ankle!); many women share the same anxiety about their pins. Don't worry, we have lots of style tips to make your legs look gorgeous, and make you feel much better about them.

Quick Fix If you are feeling vulnerable and desperate because you hate your legs, there is always safety in opaque tights! But seriously, a heel makes every leg look longer.

FEET

Whatever shape or size your feet are, we have been able to find solutions for all your feet issues. Different shaped shoes will have different effects on how you feel, and ultimately how your legs look. Remember: everyone looks better in a heel. Just break your feet in slowly with a couple of inches and slowly go higher!

Quick Fix When choosing a high heel always ensure that where your heel sits in the shoe is parallel to the ground, to ensure comfort. Anything higher puts too much pressure on the ball of your foot.

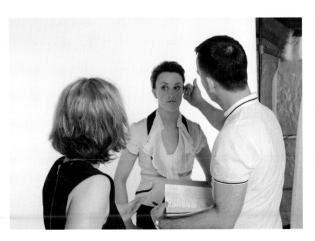
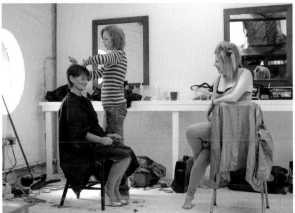

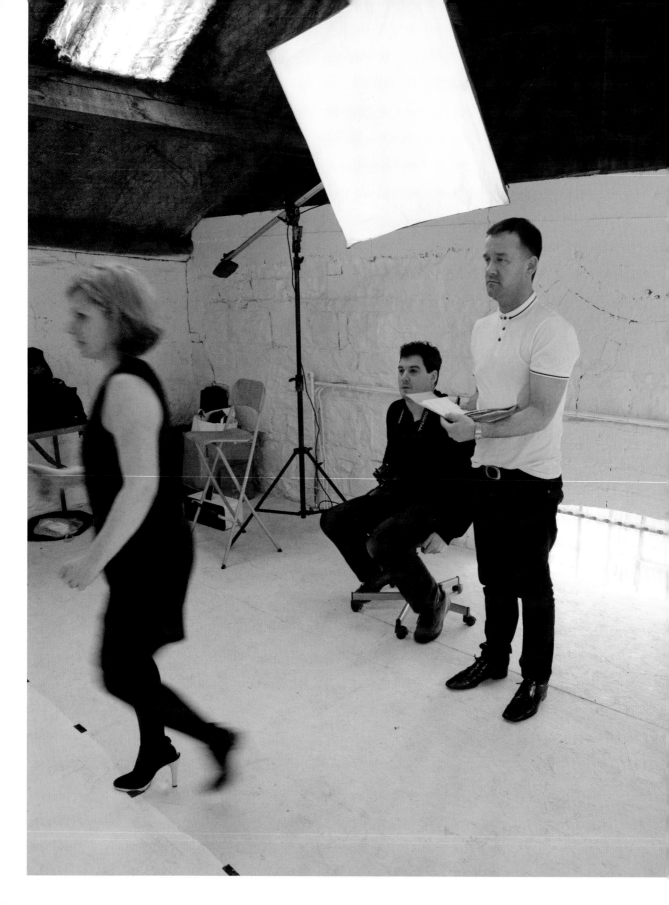

We once met a woman who wouldn't smile because when she was a little girl her teacher told her she had terrible teeth. This woman was in her forties, and had not smiled properly since childhood. We spent a very short time with her, and just got her to look in the mirror and see her teeth. We discovered that not only were they fine, but they were actually nice, and the smile that had disappeared in her childhood left the room with her that day. What people say to us as children can have a huge affect on our confidence. There are so many products on the market to improve the look of your teeth, but remember everyone looks better with a smile!

Quick Fix Even if you are not a smoker – smokers' toothpaste is amazing for stain removal!

SKIN

Your skin requires different care at different stages of your life. We will deal with this in more detail later in the book. Remember – whatever stage in life, everyone needs a daily moisturiser with minimum sun protection factor (SPF) 15 against UVA and UVB rays. The sun does untold damage to our skin and is the main perpetrator for premature aging. As we don't live in a very sunny climate, most Irish women tend to have fantastic skin right through their lives.

Quick Fix The best think you can do for your skin is to get plenty of sleep, drink lots of water and work out! But if that's too hard, maintenance through facials and good skin care definitely helps.

HAIR

Everyone needs a good hairdresser! We suggest you find a good one and cultivate mutual trust (it helps if you actually like each other). Your hair should be your crowning glory, and if you have the time – and can afford it – we would recommend visiting your hairdresser a minimum of six times a year.

Quick Fix Your hair needs to be loved and cared for, as with the rest of you, so indulge in some pampering in the form of a good treatment every now and again!

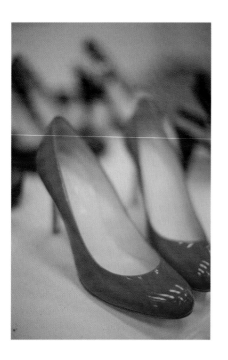

Identify what you can love about yourself

So, we've asked you to coldly list the bits of your body that you don't like. Some of you have told us that you are positively repulsed by parts of your own body. Frankly, that's not really fair on your poor body, which is only doing the best it can. The point is you've bought this book because you want to improve the way you look, and feel better about yourself. And this is the moment that the shift can begin. We bet it was really easy to identify those physical bugbears. This next bit may not come as quickly. We want you to really think about your assets. List them. How's that list shaping up? We thought so, it's not that easy on your own.

Below is a list of physical attributes that we believe to be the Irish women's natural assets. We may not have been born with French women's naturally fine legs or Italian women's naturally olive and even complexion, but Irish ladies have a lot of wonderful assets.

SO TO UNEARTH YOUR HIDDEN ASSETS HERE'S A SIMPLE EXERCISE Get your magic underwear and your new bra on, and pull those straps good and tight (instant boob lift). Now put on a slip or body suit. Forget it's you in the mirror and take a long hard look, only this time with your 'glass half full' head on. Ask your style buddy for help with this, some fresh eyes are exactly what's required here.

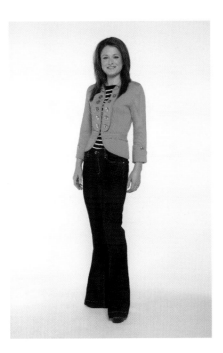

The things you should be looking out for are listed below. If you find assets that we haven't thought of – brilliant!

OUR NATURAL ASSETS

- Luminous skin
- Radiant eyes
- Great boobs
- Thick hair
- Youthful décolletage
- Delicious curves (forget about child-bearing hips and think Marilyn Monroe)
- Wit and charm (You're Irish, after all!)
- Smile to die for (The minute you start to harness your own power, trust us, this will be your sexiest feature. Nothing is sexier than a confident woman.)
- Good legs (if you're fixating on your belly, you may not even realise they exist)
- Your neck
- Your clavicle (collarbone)
- The narrowest point on your torso (often just below the bust line).

Does anything in there tickle your fancy? Try and forget it's you in the mirror, and see if that works. The power to look good begins in your head, you must realise that wallowing in dissatisfaction with your body is pointless. So, now, what do you see?

Pick three assets to focus on, and as your confidence grows, the albatross of your bum/belly/hips (insert as appropriate!) can fade into the background. In chapter 6, we give you all the practical advice you need to best display your assets and conceal your bugbears. Check our photographic guide of real women being taught how to tackle their real body issues.

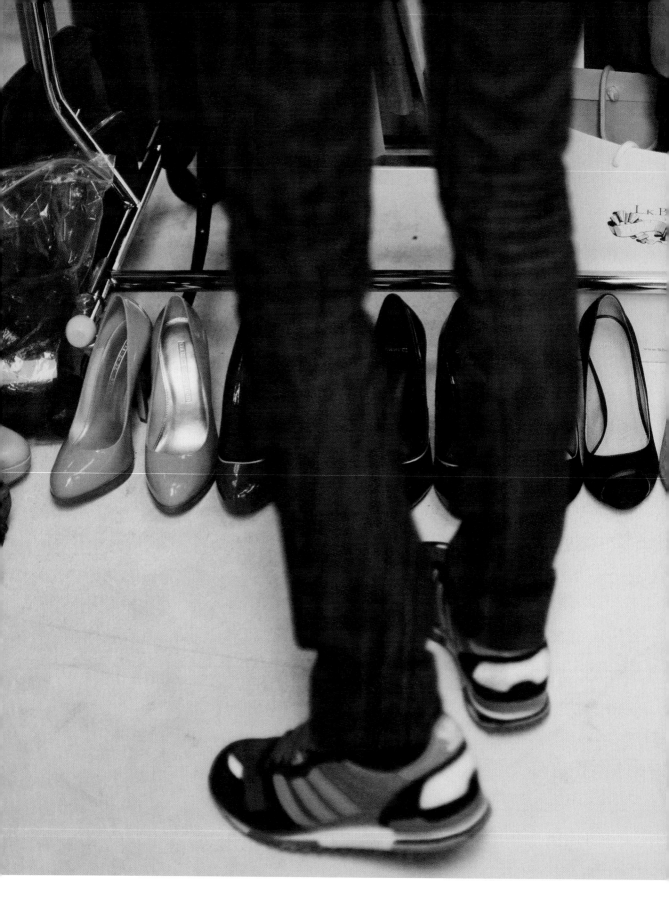

chapter four

THE IMPORTANCE OF WEARING THE RIGHT SIZE BRA

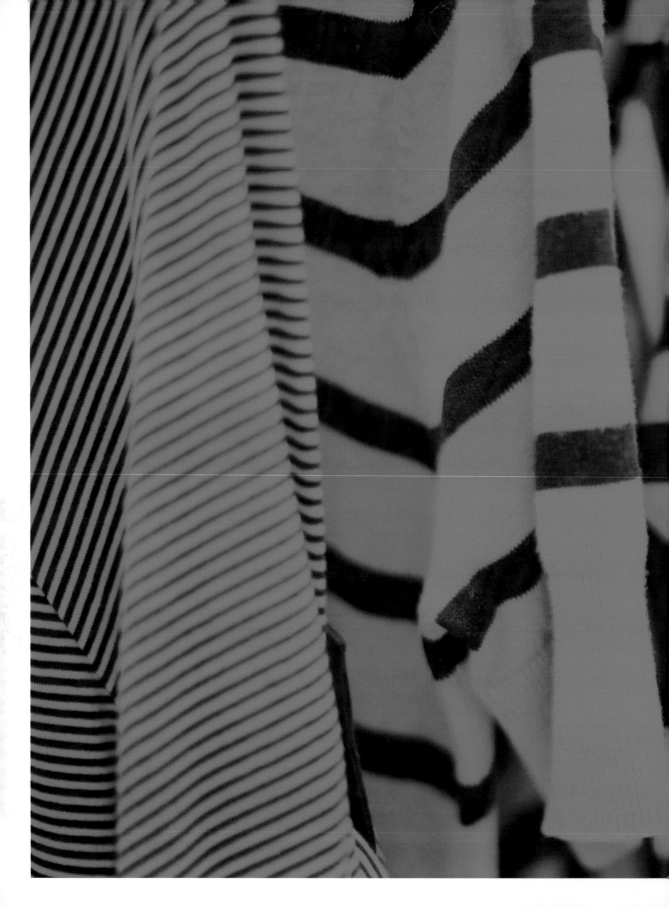

When we started OFF THE RAILS, because of our backgrounds, we thought we would be well prepared for any situation, particularly the underwear situation, and thought that the fact that a lot of women wear the wrong size bra would not phase us. But nothing could have prepared us for the scale of the problem – literally every single woman we have worked with has been wearing the wrong size bra! We realised that this problem was pandemic, and so took it upon ourselves to do the first ever 'OFF THE RAILS National Bra Fitting Day', in November 2008. We took over the window of Clery's department store, on O'Connell St, Dublin, and had all the fabulous women who showed up re-measured. The reaction to that day was so big that we felt 'wearing the right bra size', deserves its own chapter.

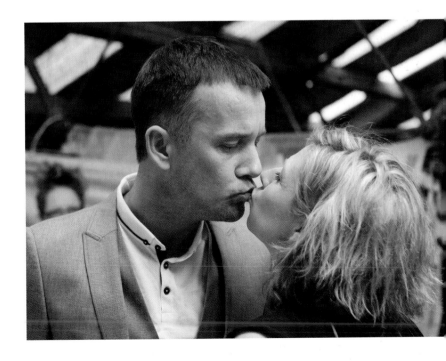

Why are we wearing the wrong size bra?

First off girls it is okay, this is not a scolding! Don't panic, nearly every woman wears the wrong size bra and here's why:

- Shockingly, some shops will sell you what they have in stock, as opposed to your actual size. Certainly not all shops but it does happen.
- Using an unqualified or inexperienced measurer.
- Women's bodies can change as often as monthly, but few women change their bras to reflect this.
- Your bra is supposed to be tight (not uncomfortable), but tight, nonetheless.
- Wearing the same bra for years!

So why is it so important to wear the correct size bra?

To answer in three words: support, silhouette and confidence.

The most obvious reason is support. For lift and hold we need to put those bad boys in their right place and hold them there. No matter what the size, they need to be lifted and held, then everything underneath becomes streamlined and much easier to dress. Here's the science girls – the primary support from a well-fitting bra comes from the back strap, in our experience women tend to wear bras at least two inches too big on the back.

Once your boobs are in the right place your silhouette is instantly improved and your back is better protected.

Confidence is the greatest benefit of wearing the correct bra size and underwear – you will feel instantly supported, like you have your own cheerleading team under your clothes supporting you! Your clothes sit and fit 100 per cent better, and so your body shape is reconstructed in an instant. In our makeovers, this is the area that always surprises and amazes our ladies the most, and where the transformation really starts to happen.

Before 38D

Problem: Back size too big, cup size too small and shoulder straps too loose.

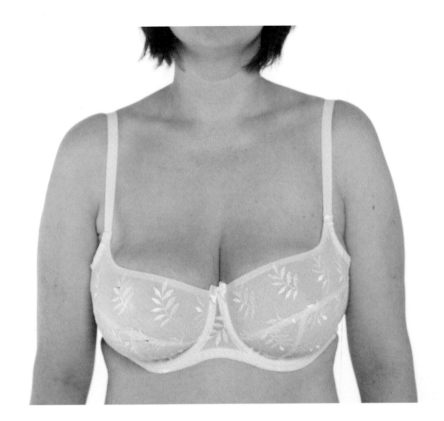

After 34F

Solution: Correct back size – gives correct back support. Central panel sitting flush against breast bone. Full cup support, eliminating the risk of 'double boob'. Straps tight for max lift and control.

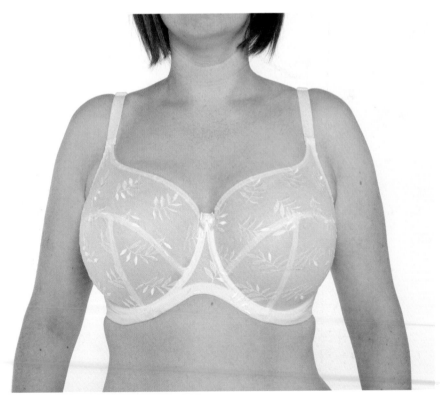

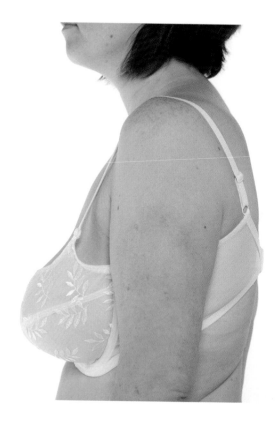

Before 38D
*The first point of support is
the back strap.*

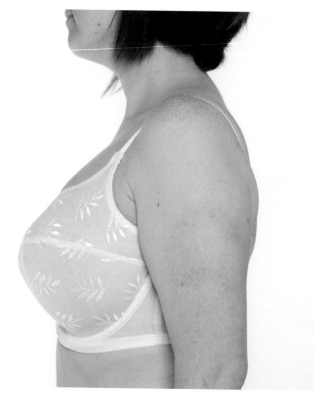

After 34F
*The correct back size and
cup size will also guarantee
improved posture.*

It's that simple girl – when you have the right size bra on, you look and feel great. Your clothes look and feel so much better.

So, invest wisely in the basics, as it makes more economic sense in the long run. Even the best clothing around will look rubbish over the wrong size bra.

HOW IT WORKS

To understand what the right size bra means, you should know that the primary support is coming from the back strap. Nothing will work if the back strap's not right. Secondary support comes from the cup, and last, but not least your bra straps give you that all important lift.

How to make sure you are wearing the right size bra

1. The size you measure on the measuring tape, is not necessarily the size you should wear; it takes an experienced and qualified bra fitter to determine your correct size bra. They will get you to try on a few sizes, until you find the right one for you.

2. Get measured regularly – it only takes two minutes – women's bodies are fabulous creations and change all the time. It's the wonderful thing about being a woman. We suggest every woman should get re-measured regularly, but especially after the following: losing weight, gaining weight, toning up, during pregnancy, post baby, post breast feeding, starting the pill, coming off the pill, or any kind of back injury.

3. Ideally a bra that fits properly should sit flush to the breastbone.

4. When buying a new bra – bring a t-shirt along, so you can see clearly if the bra fits correctly.

Note It is recommended that women avoid wearing underwire bras during pregnancy and breastfeeding, as it can interfere with the changes in a woman's breasts.

5. As we've said, most women wear their bras too big on the back. When you come down a back size, you automatically go up a cup size. For example, a woman who was a 36B becomes a delicious 34C, nice eh?

6. If you find that the straps of the bra are digging into your shoulders, it is because the back is too big. If the back is not firm enough, it will cause the straps to dig in and give ridges – therefore always make sure the back is firm and not too loose.

7. Spillage – if the cup is too small, this causes the breasts to spill out of the bra and instead of two beautiful breasts, you end up looking like you have four boobs – not a good look!

8. Always start a new bra on the loosest clasps, that means as the bra starts to age and stretch, you can make it last longer, by moving up a clasp, to keep it taut and firm.

INSTANT HIT

Take a look at your bra right now, and for an instant lift, tighten the bra straps, you will see an immediate improvement. You should tighten your bra straps every day. If you think about it, it makes total sense; you wouldn't walk around with your skirt not closed properly, or (we hope) your knickers at your knees!

We cannot stress enough how important it is to wear the right size bra ladies, so go out now and get yourself re-measured and start to actually change the way you support, dress, and ultimately, see your body.

Before 38D
Problem: Straps are too loose and incorrect back size.

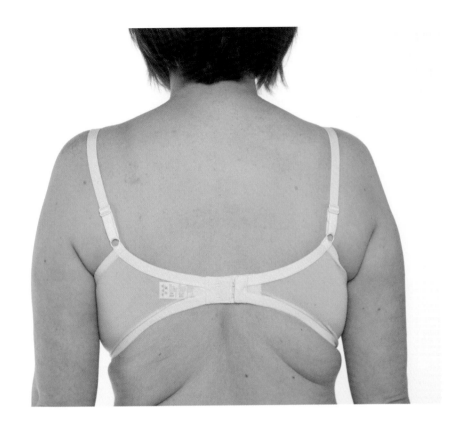

Before 34F
Solution: Correct back size, cupsize and straps are nice and taut.

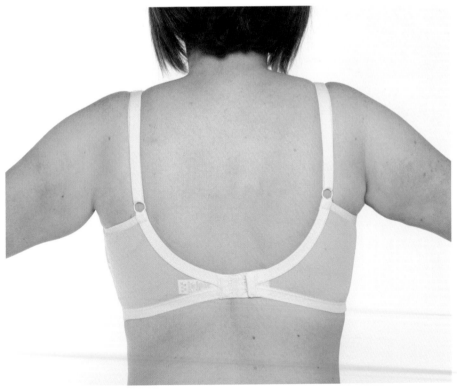

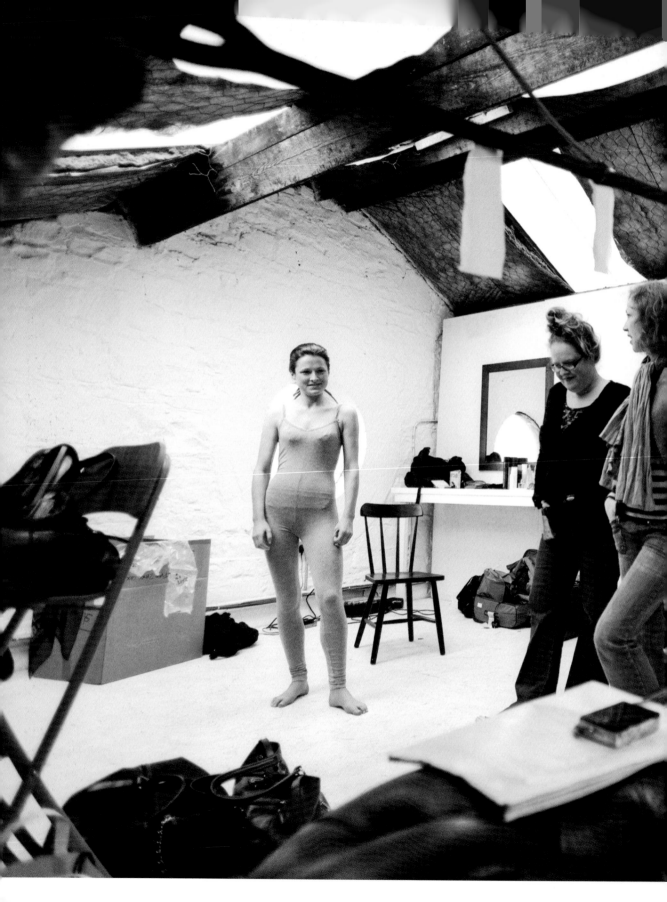

5

EVERYTHING YOU ALWAYS WANTED TO KNOW ABOUT SHAPEWEAR BUT WERE AFRAID TO ASK

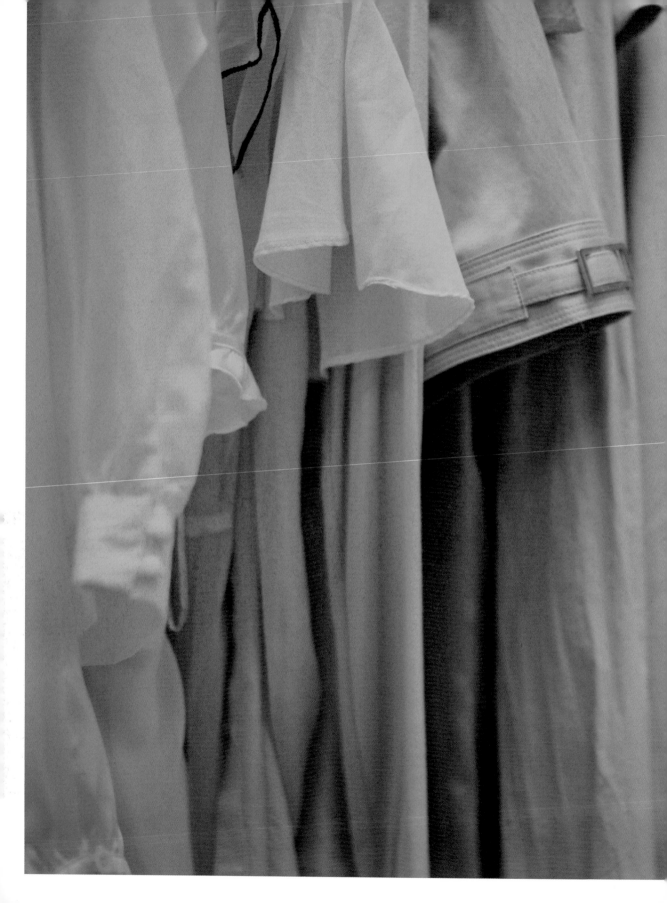

No matter what your shape (Apple, Pear or even Ruler), there is a shapewear garment out there to help you. Shapewear is still a mystical world to many of you. It can be very intimidating to the uninitiated. Most of it looks ugly and uncomfortable. It is also very easy to buy the wrong garment for your shape, leading to costly mistakes.

So why bother pouring yourself into what looks like an instrument of torture? We have found that, regardless of your shape and size, there is shapewear out there that will make you feel more confident about how you look. And for us, and you, that is the bottom line (excuse the pun). Once you try a little bit of this magic, we think you'll understand why we're so passionate about its power. In this chapter, we try to untangle the mystery of shapewear and offer you valuable tips for its use. We are not suggesting that it becomes part of your everyday armour, but rather a tool to build your confidence in your own power to look good.

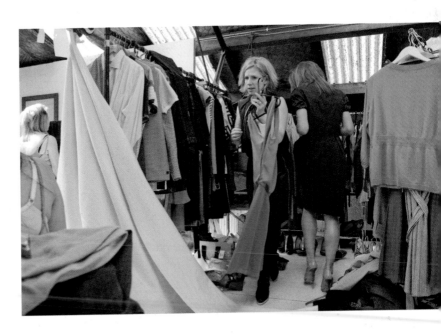

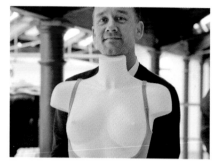

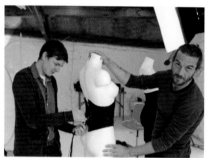

How to pick the right shapewear

Women can have a collection of shapewear according to its function, and the garment it's being worn under. Relate your shapewear garment to what you're going to wear over it – this is important. It's only magic if you don't know it's there.

What is 'spillage'

The controlling nature of these creations can lead to the risk of 'spillage'. What is 'spillage'? Spillage is the point at which the controlling power of shapewear stops, and the force of your body takes over, resulting in unsightly lumps and bumps. Let's talk about the garment that you're going to be wearing. If you've opted for a brave diva number, which skims all your fabulous curves – firstly, Bravo! That's the spirit! Secondly, you have to choose your shapewear accordingly. Each different type of shapewear has a specific job to do. See below, for a beginners' guide on how to choose what's right for you.

SHAPEWEAR THONG CONTROLOMETER ★★

The shapewear thong is a light control garment. Ideal for women whose only issue is a little belly bump. These are readily available from most lingerie departments. The ideal usage would be to smooth out the tummy for a fitted skirt or trousers. If the garment worn on top is very fitted, you run the risk of an unsightly line being visible at the waist.

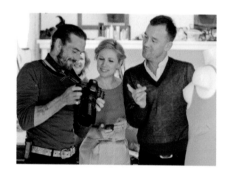

SHAPEWEAR PANTS CONTROLOMETER ★★★

Not everyone can handle the thong, and in lingerie terms it's no longer that fashionable, having been replaced by shorties or bigger more feminine shapes. Dita Von Teese has a lot to answer for. If you need tummy support and don't want a thong, then shapewear pants are for you. Again, if you have an issue with your thighs, these are not for you, as you will get 'spillage'.

SHAPEWEAR KNICKERS CONTROLOMETER ★★★★

If the area you need to control extends from your belly to your thighs, then shapewear knickers are for you. Again, the possibility of spillage above the waist is high. But, these bad boys do a very important job, they wrangle all the way down to mid thigh.

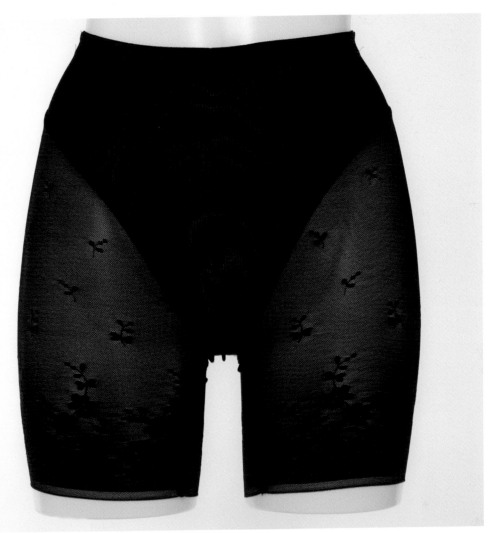

Shapewear knickers

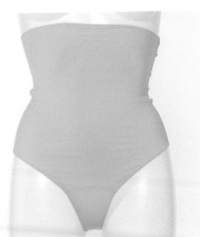

Shapewear thong

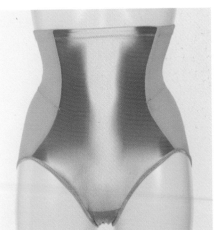

Shapewear pants

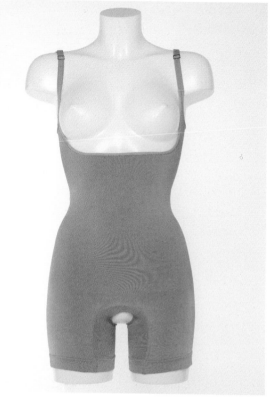

Shapewear body

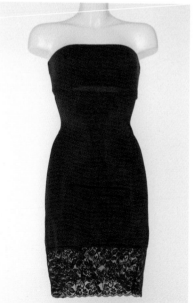

Shapewear body thong

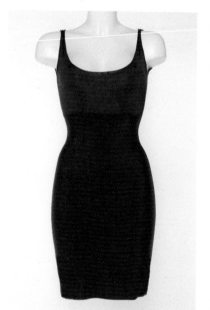

Shapewear slip

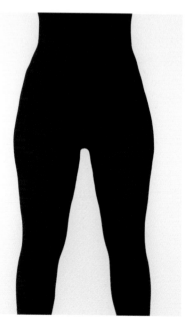

Shapewear strapless slip

Shapewear control leggings

SHAPEWEAR BODY CONTROLOMETER ★★★★★

This is shapewear at full force. We use a shapewear body on most of our transformation candidates. The reason being that it offers full body, seamless support, regardless of the look that we choose for our lovely lady. If you have an unforgiving fitted dress, this is the one for you.

The shapewear body works so well, primarily because the straps keep it firmly in place. Some strapless shapewear create the dreaded roll and shift, which has you running to the loo to fix yourself every ten minutes, not a good look.

SHAPEWEAR BODY THONG CONTROLOMETER ★★★

A sexier version of this, without the thigh support, is the shapewear body thong. It doesn't have the intense power of its sister, but you'll be proud to reveal this little number.

SHAPEWEAR SLIP CONTROLOMETER ★★★★★

The shapewear slip is the more feminine sister of the shapewear body. It performs the same function but is only for use under skirts and dresses, as it doesn't have thigh-hugging legs. The benefit of this is that the ugly spectre of the open gusset is avoided. However, there is a risk of the shapewear skirt rolling and moving slightly. Look for a rubber runner on the inside of the hem, this will help to keep it in place. It's important not to use talc or body creams, as this will stop the rubber trim from doing its job.

Also available in this category is a strapless version for your red carpet moment or a balmy evening.

WAIST CINCHER CONTROLOMETER ★★

The waist cincher gives great light support. Essentially, it gives definition to a smaller frame – it is great for Rulers. Again, if you need all-over control this is not for you, as it will produce spillage top and bottom.

CONTROL LEGGINGS CONTROLOMETER ★★

Control leggings are like thick tights, they reduce the appearance of cellulite and give bums and thighs the

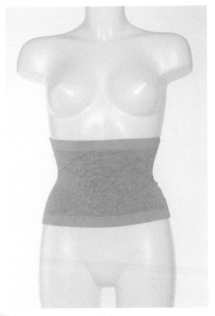

Shapewear waist cincher

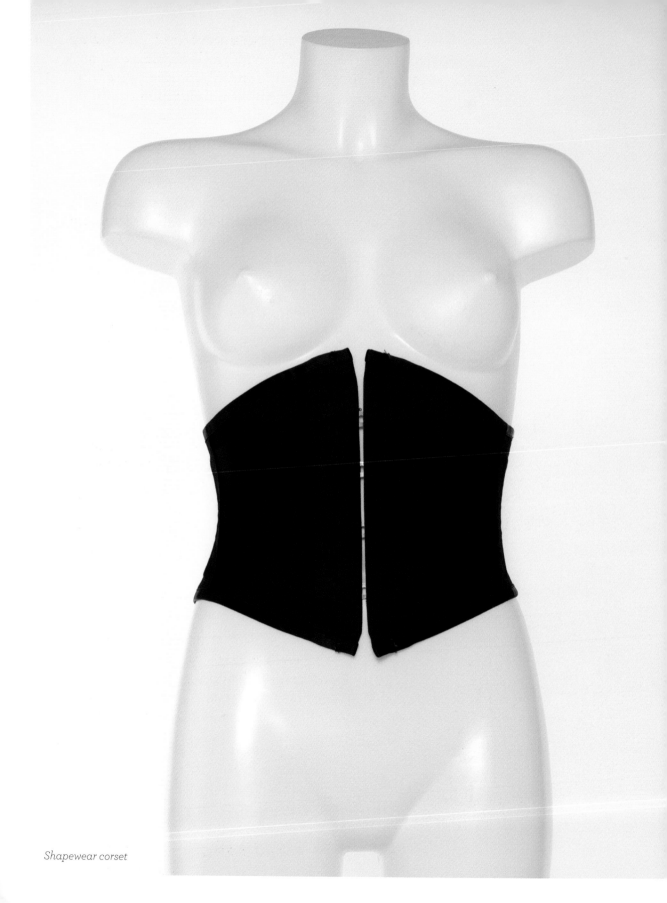

Shapewear corset

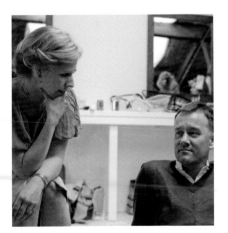

same support and control as shapewear pants. They are a great confidence booster for you ladies who want to attempt skinny jeans. A commonly available alternative of these, are their lighter cousin, control tights.

CORSET

The original and sexiest version of shapewear is the corset. Apart from the obvious, the benefit of this garment is that it will make you feel like a Hollywood siren. Unfortunately, boning and lacing mean that this garment is not always possible to conceal, however, if you own one, you may not want to.

How do I go to the toilet? Generally, shapewear is designed with a semi-open gusset, which you manoeuver to allow yourself to go to the toilet. The cleverer (and often more expensive) ones come with popper studs.

Indecent exposure? Many of you are appalled by the concept of an essentially open gusset, and feel that it is not a practical solution. We agree! However, that is where design has brought us to date. We feel sure that progress can only be around the corner.

Please don't be tempted to wear your own underwear underneath as a layer of protection. This will create knicker lines, which is the very thing that shapewear is created to avoid.

Our main piece of advice about shape and control underwear is to simply give it a try. We have yet to put it on somebody who hasn't been dazzled by its effects. And remember, you don't have to wear them all the time, but for that little bit of a confidence boost, they could turn out to be your new best friend.

Leabharlanna Poibli Chathair Bhaile Átha Cliath
Dublin City Public Libraries

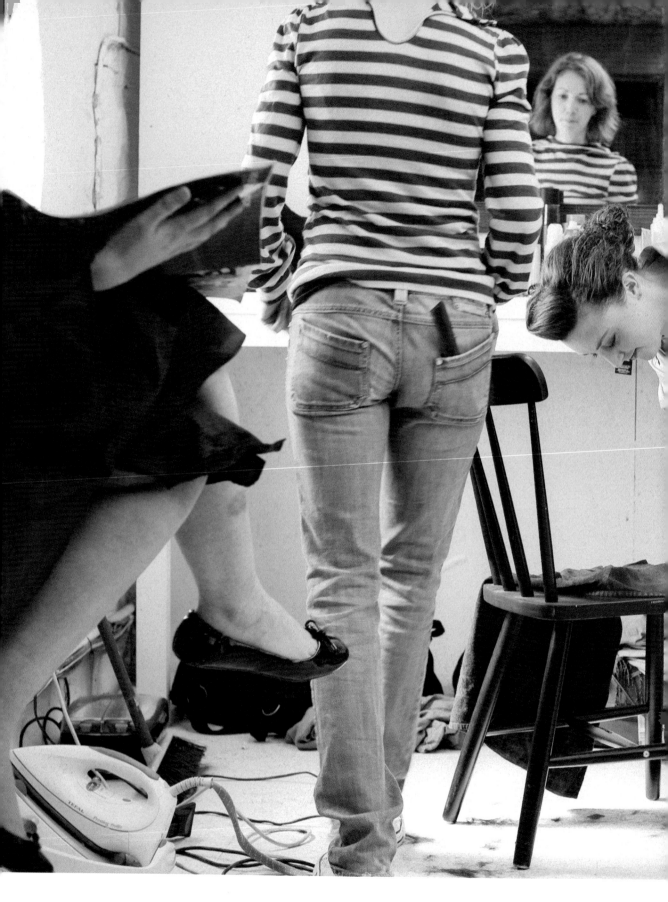

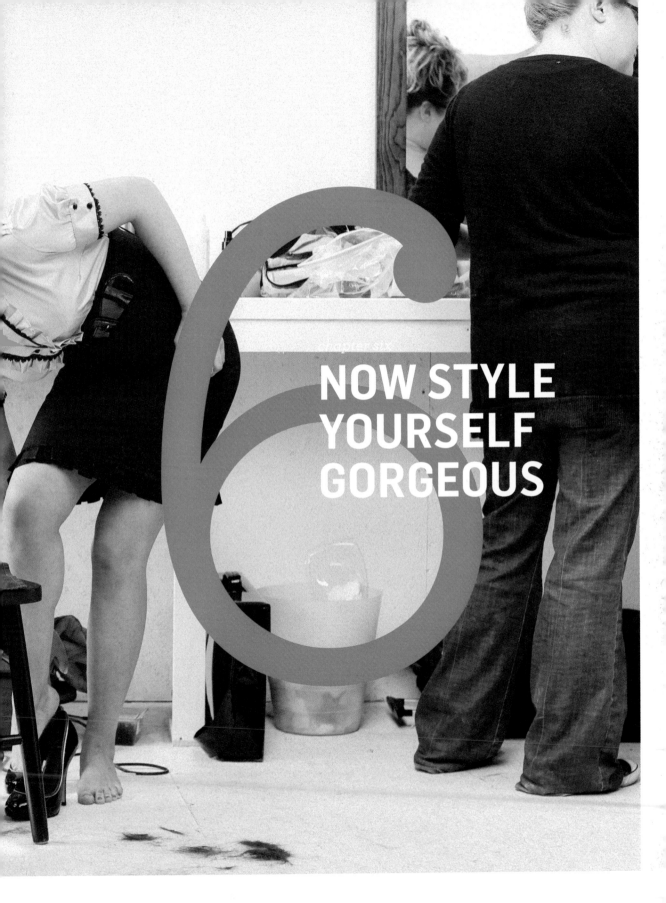

chapter six

NOW STYLE YOURSELF GORGEOUS

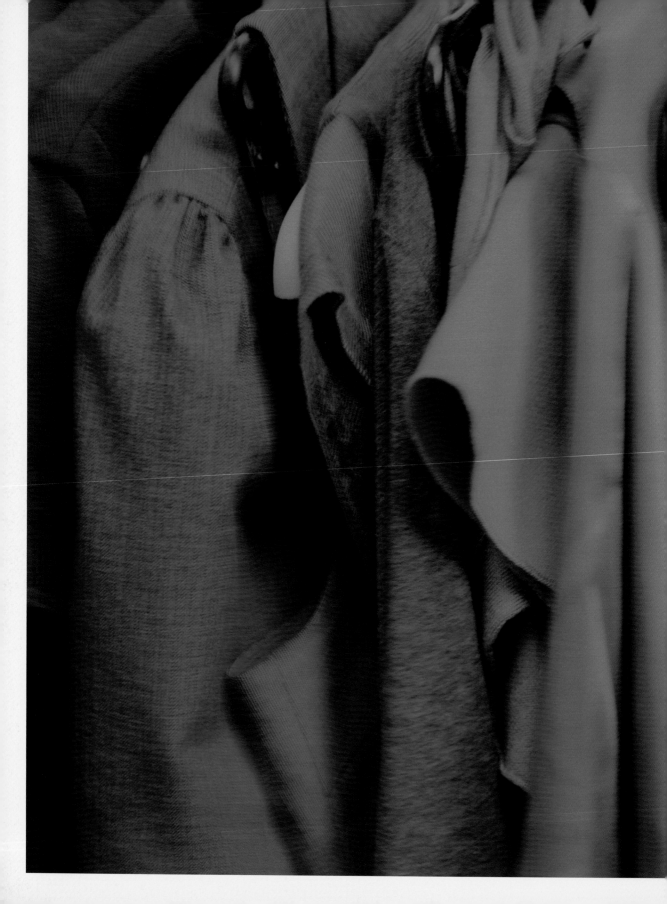

Now that you have identified your body shape and have seen the benefits of wearing the right underwear, this chapter shows you simple ways to look great for any occasion, from a trip to the supermarket to a hot date.

We have deliberately kept the styling very simple and uncluttered in these photographs. These looks are a guide to understanding how clothes can change the silhouette of our bodies. Consider this as an exercise in the basic principles of body architecture.

The looks that we have chosen are based on classic styles and are not trend driven. We believe that all of the items shown will give you years of style and represent the basic building blocks of a fully functioning wardrobe.

Classic style is ageless and timeless. To show the broad appeal of our collection, we did a little experiment. We took two gorgeous Petite ladies, Michelle, in her twenties, and Deirdre, in her forties, and gave them the same two outfits to try on. We think you'll agree that the looks work on both women and that they look equally chic and sexy.

We've picked four key looks for every woman's needs. Nail these, and you will have the foundations of a fully functioning wardrobe. These four looks are solutions to the areas of difficulty which so many of you have encountered.

The four key looks

COMFORT CHIC (DOWN TIME)

This is a new way to approach feeling good while doing the most day-to-day chores. Supermarket shopping or doing the school run need not be a style-less activity. In fact, why not make looking good one less thing to worry about? We'll let you hold onto your tracksuit for when you've got the flu, but try to get that invigorating style injection during the most routine tasks, and you will start your style addiction, which will grow and develop from there.

WORK TO PLAY (DAY TO NIGHT)

'Dress for the job you want, not for the job you have'
Even if you're not a career girl, this great multi-functioning look is designed to help you move seamlessly from day to night with confidence, comfort and style.

SHOPPING (LUNCH WITH THE GIRLS)

This is all about optimum daytime chic, cranking up the style dial without going too high glamour. It can be a tricky one to get right, but with our fool-proof approach, don't worry ladies, you'll nail it.

OH MY GOD! (SHE LOOKS AMAZING!)

Whatever the occasion, 'occasion wear' trips up so many women. The country is full of wardrobes with once worn outfits that were panic bought for a special occasion and then despised for the rest of their lives. It doesn't have to be so. Buy cleverly and your best pieces can take you from a posh dinner to a wedding reception.

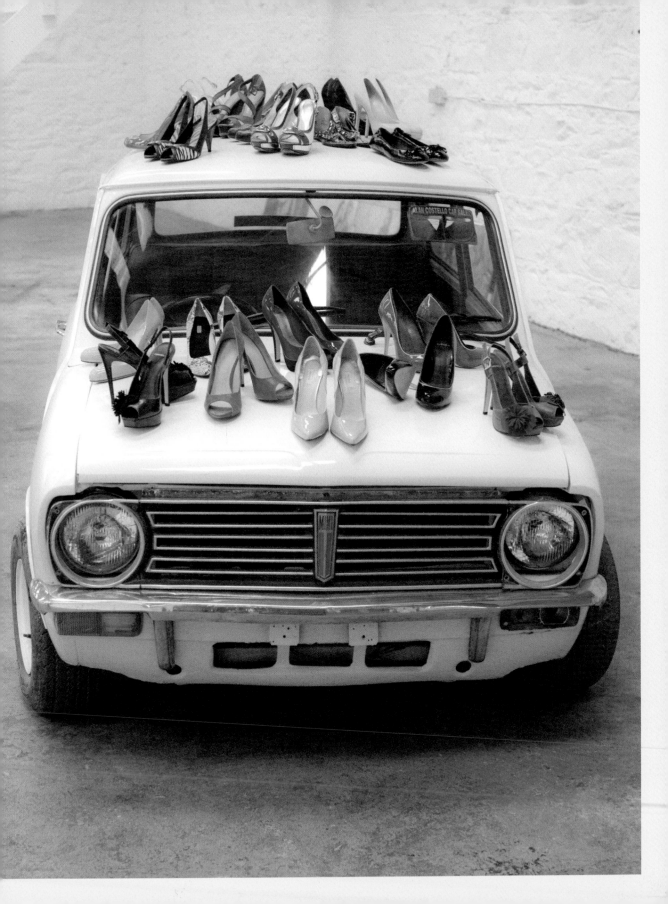

AFTER
STREAMLINED PEAR

Correct bra size
The correct sized bra lifts and supports.

Shapewear
Nadia is getting maximum support
for her tummy and thighs.

PEAR

BEFORE

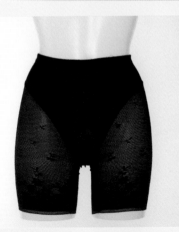

Opposite:
Nadia is wearing shapewear knickers

For our wonderful pears this is what we suggest you aim for and what you should avoid.

Mantra

- Play to your strengths and focus on your top half
- Find the beauty in softer, flowing and draped fabrics that skim the hips
- Highlight your waist with structure and balance with a fuller skirt
- Use detailing and embellishment on your top half, to draw the eye up
- It's all about using the shoulders to create balance
- Go for high-waisted jeans with a wide leg in indigo or dark dye. Don't crop the length, go as long as you can bear (Remember you can conceal a platform shoe under there to further lengthen the body)

Avoid

- Tight fitting fabrics
- Hip pockets, pleats and embellishment on the hip area or around your middle
- Over emphasising your tiny waist (it will make your hips seem bigger), unless you create that all important balance with a fuller skirt
- Never try to hide in baggy clothes – it will always make you look much larger
- Clingy fabrics on your lower half
- Ankle straps

Comfort chic (down time)

You now know your perfect jeans shape. The same applies to trousers. Define the waist, skim the hips and wear the hem long, to maximise your shape. Remember to keep your lower half in darker tones (and you know we don't just mean black!), which are more slimming on your shape. But go as wild as you like with colour and embellishment on top. This gorgeous coral colour is one of our favourites for wearability and sheer feel-good factor. Notice how the shoulder line is gently extended with soft pleating to balance the silhouette.

Team this look with a classic trench or cropped fitted jacket for chic appeal.

Brilliant news, this autumn marks the return of your new best friend – the shoulder pad! Mainly associated with the '80s, this useful item is excellent for balance and thanks to the international catwalks, super stylish. Think structure when it comes to jackets, wide lapels with nipped in waist, will give you diva-like proportions (jackets should end no lower than top of the hip).

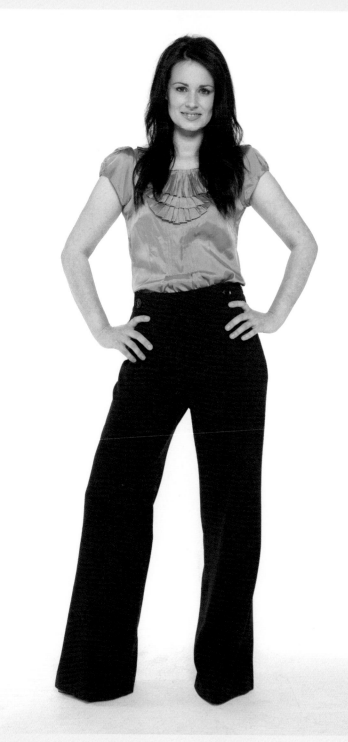

COMFORT CHIC

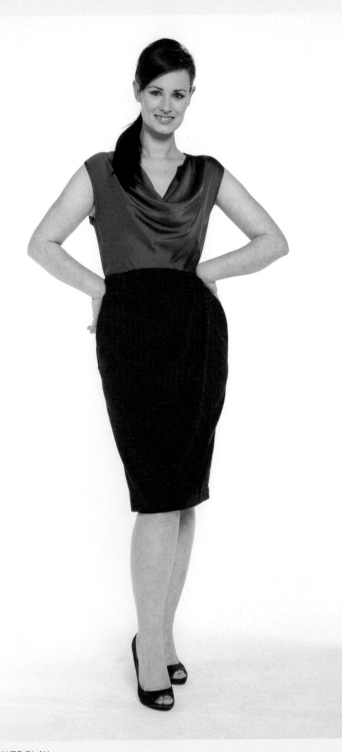

This little bit of fashion magic looks like a two-piece, but is actually a dress. So, the ease of one garment, with the benefits of a skirt and top. This allows you to get your colour fix on your top half and, in the case of this version, gently swathe your curves in a soft black crepe. The clever wrap detailing is perfect for your shape, because it breaks up the lower half and, as it comes in below the knee, it draws the eye down to your fabulous shoes.

This dress is probably the best way for a pear to tackle 'figure hugging'. The soft drape of the top, and gentle overhang of the shoulder means the waist is not overemphasised, and creates the beautiful balance of an hour-glass silhouette.

Go to work in a full-skirted coat, which would be perfect over this dress, giving classic femininity and definition. Whip it off for night-time, and for instant outfit upgrade – add a chunky statement necklace to keep the eye at your top half.

WORK TO PLAY

Shopping (lunch with the girls)

Nothing is more enduring than the style of a Hitchcock heroine; luckily for you it's your optimum silhouette. Now this is what we're talking about, the fuller skirt cleverly conceals the hips, while the tailored top and pretty shoulder generate balance.

The perfect balance of this dress is completed with a pretty flat pump. If you want to drive this look home, a feminine embellished cardigan would be super-cute or throw in a curveball with a harder edged denim cropped jacket.

Oh my God! (She looks amazing!)

For evening wear it is always nice to reveal a little skin. Importantly this is also all about balance, the balance between reveal and conceal. So, lovely pear, reveal your slender top half and gently drape your lower half. Interestingly, the eye sees the narrowness on show, and assumes that the same proportions continue under the fabric. This is the magic of volume when used correctly. Technically, this dress shouldn't work, because it's in such a pale coral, and yet the cleverness of the drape and cut mean that it works perfectly on Nadia's proportions.

This brings us back to our primary lesson – always try it on!

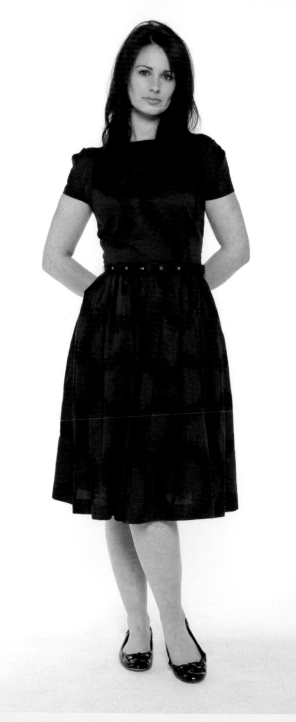

LUNCH WITH THE GIRLS

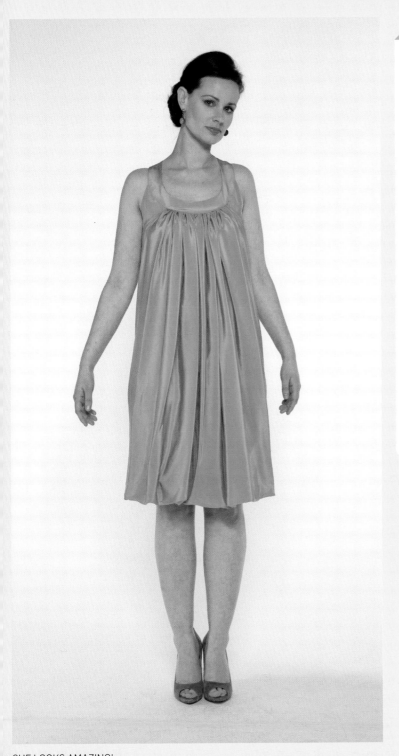

SHE LOOKS AMAZING!

Accessories

- Bags should be worn underarm (never worn or carried at hip height, because it will make the area appear bigger).

- Statement jewellery – go mad, you can wear big stuff up top. That means earrings and necklaces, but no bracelets or rings. Also no loud or low slung belts, as they will draw attention to your hips!

- Try to get to grips with a good court shoe, as it always makes the leg look longer than a shoe cut higher on the front of the foot.

- During the winter, a pair of riding boots is a great staple. Just make sure that your skirt length covers the top of the boots, to elongate the line of the body.

AFTER
STREAMLINED APPLE

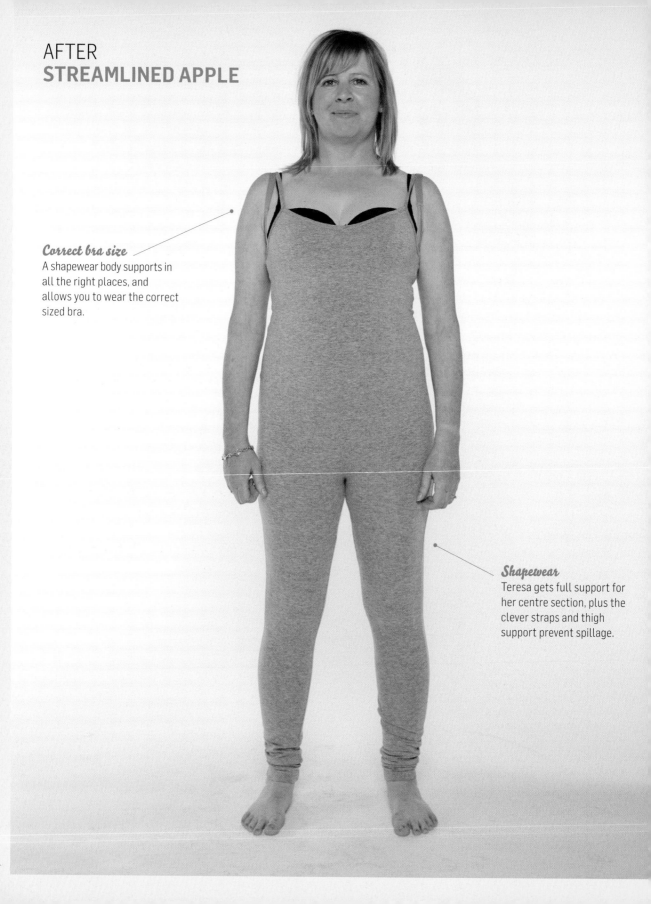

Correct bra size
A shapewear body supports in all the right places, and allows you to wear the correct sized bra.

Shapewear
Teresa gets full support for her centre section, plus the clever straps and thigh support prevent spillage.

APPLE

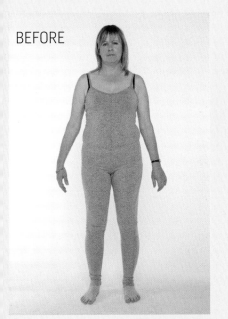

For our delicious apples, here are our basic principles to dressing your shape.

Mantra

- Use tailoring and colour to define and reshape your torso
- Highlight and create a waist (it's easy!) – fabulous belts are your new best friend, when worn at your narrowest point
- Get your legs and arms out
- V and scoop neck everything, to lengthen the neck and draw the eye to that gorgeous cleavage

Avoid

- Baggy clothing – it doesn't disguise anything and only makes you look much bigger
- Shapeless shift dresses
- Anything double breasted which will just bulk you out at your mid section

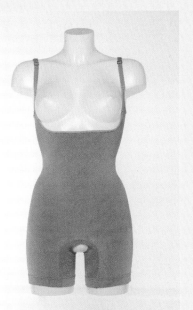

Opposite:
Teresa is wearing a shapewear body

Comfort chic (down time)

You may not believe this, but there are jeans for you. Try boot cut or parallel (trousers that are the same width at the hip as at the hem) first, then advance to wide leg, but remember to stay neat on that slim thigh. This will add volume and balance to your lower half, thus making your waist look smaller. Wear them all the way to the floor with heeled boots, for maximum leg length-ening affect.

Add a single-breasted fitted jacket or structured knit that closes just under your boobs to finish off the creation. Voila – your new waist! Remember that the aim of the jacket is to create and define your waist. So pay attention to where its hemline hits, if it sits lower than your natural waist, make sure that it hugs to the waist and falls out in a skirted or frilled detail.

Empire line tops add a little volume again to make the waist appear smaller. For our lovely ap-ples, a wrap top is the perfect partner for so many looks.

Now have fun, try a figure-defining waistcoat – we promise you, you won't look back!

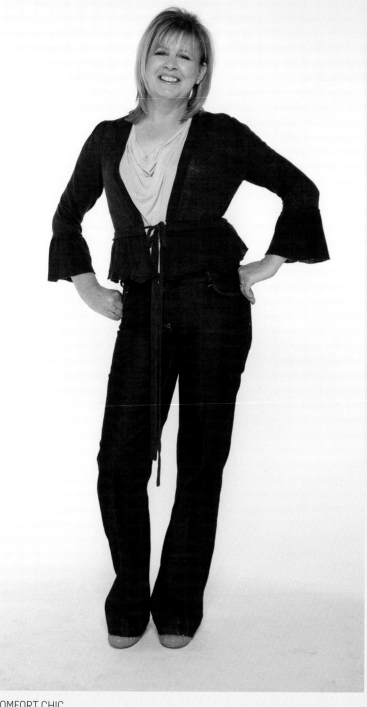

COMFORT CHIC

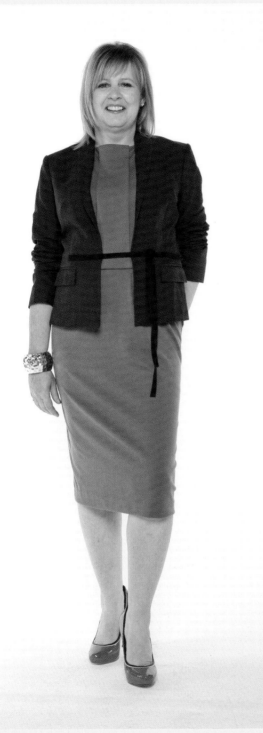

Building up the palette for Teresa's new wardrobe, we introduced her to this beautiful soft mushroom shade, which is gorgeous on her colouring. The supportive stretch jersey and clever cut of this classic dress makes it a must-have for any apple. Soft pleating below the waistband narrows the mid section. Add to the mix this clever tailored jacket with narrow belting and you've got a winning look.

Most people would say Apples can't wear pencil skirts! We don't agree, every woman should have a sexy pencil skirt, and this dress is a good starting point. Go on give it a go!

WORK TO PLAY

Shopping (lunch with the girls)

Clever tailoring can never be overestimated for you – this well chosen tailored jacket cinches in the waist and gives definition to the upper body. Some volume on the skirt creates hips. Add into the mix a central pleat, and hey presto – a curvy elongated silhouette! Using the jacket as an accessory and leaving it open slices the mid section, and draws the eye in and up. Everything about this outfit points to a tiny waist.

Also try a wraparound dress with deep V. This will break up the width of your torso. Add a camisole underneath to create interest and depth, or be brave and enjoy your cleavage. A chic and clever way to draw attention to those pins is to have some fun with coloured tights.

Oh my God! (She looks amazing!)

Shapeless shifts and baggy dresses are an absolute no-no, but get the cut right, like this tailored pencil dress with clever capped sleeves, and you're on to a winner. Add a belt to highlight your newly discovered waist.

With the right dress, you will start to feel more confident exposing your arms and legs. You can achieve this look with a skirt and blouse too, just keep your eye-catching belt handy.

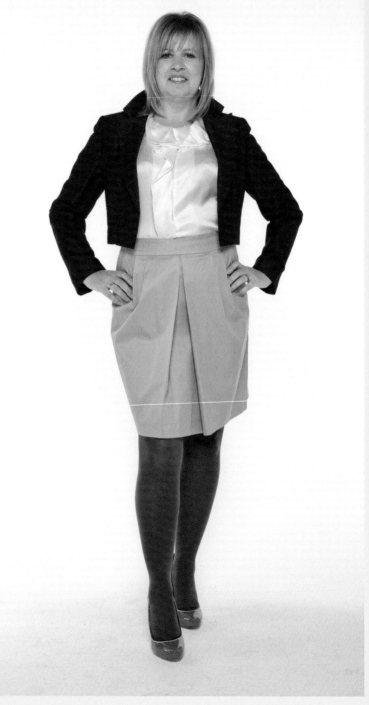

LUNCH WITH THE GIRLS

Try halter neck or even strapless dresses, and you will not only be feeling super sexy, but they will break up your torso perfectly. Remember, a high heel elongates the leg, but avoid ankle straps, as they will make the leg look shorter.

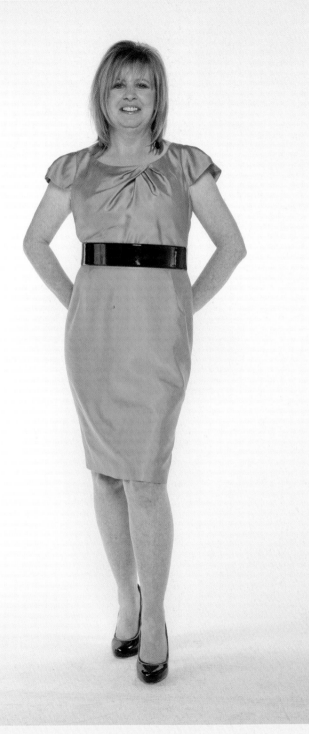

SHE LOOKS AMAZING!

Accessories

- Have fun with coloured tights; your legs are one of your best features and this is a way to get them out without getting them out!

- Belts, belts, belts: use tie-belts and let them hang down one side to have an elongating and narrowing effect on your body.

- Long scarves have a great effect on your shape.

- Go for bold statement necklaces, but avoid going too long; we want to draw the eye up, away from your mid section.

- Carry big bags over your shoulder with a short strap to stop at your newly-discovered waist; this will add to your new waist definition. Similarly, a clutch works great on you.

- Avoid strappy shoes, as they will shorten your leg. The higher the heel, the longer the leg.

- Try capped or puffed sleeves for a gorgeous feminine silhouette.

- A box jacket with shoulder pads will create balance and make your waist look more defined.

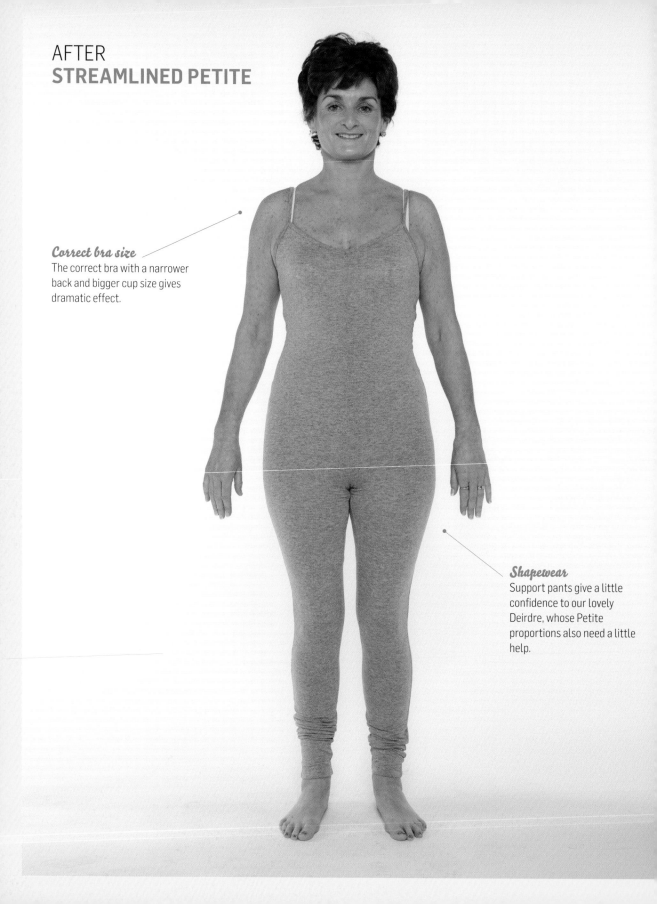

AFTER
STREAMLINED PETITE

Correct bra size
The correct bra with a narrower back and bigger cup size gives dramatic effect.

Shapewear
Support pants give a little confidence to our lovely Deirdre, whose Petite proportions also need a little help.

PETITE

Small and perfectly formed, here are your tips to looking great.

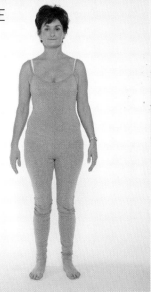

BEFORE

Mantra

- Elongate the silhouette from neck to toe
- Use one colour/tonal play
- V-necks
- Emphasise the waist
- Go for mid-calf skirts over knee-length boots
- Wedge shoes
- Use parallel trousers with high waists to lengthen the leg

Avoid

- Large patterns
- Volume in the wrong place
- Baggy, shapeless clothing

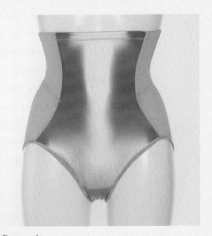

Opposite:
Deirdre is wearing shapewear pants

Comfort chic (down time)

This outfit is timeless and ageless and can be worn by women of different ages. Both Deirdre and Michelle look fantastic in this outfit.

Take a cropped jacket (we love this orange military style) and use it as a stylish outer casing for your look. If your jacket looks chic, it's amazing what you can get away with! For comfort, choose flat pumps or wedge heels. Unless you are very slim, avoid cropped trousers, as they will shorten your silhouette. Try to introduce some colour on top.

Slim cashmere knits are a really good basic that make you look and feel fabulous.

These tailored high-waisted jeans in dark denim are a fabulous staple. They look much smarter than their straight-legged pale counterparts, and can even double up for work-wear, if teamed with a delicate blouse and a nipped in jacket.

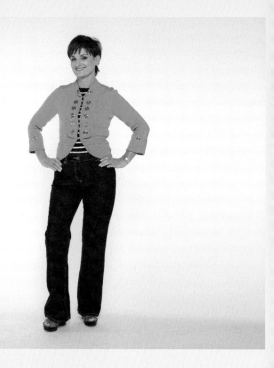

COMFORT CHIC
Deirdre, our fabulous 40-something model is chic and comfortable in this great look.

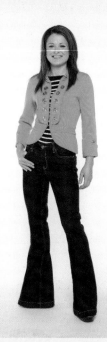

COMFORT CHIC
Michelle, our glamourous 20-something gal also works this 'timeless' outfit with ease.

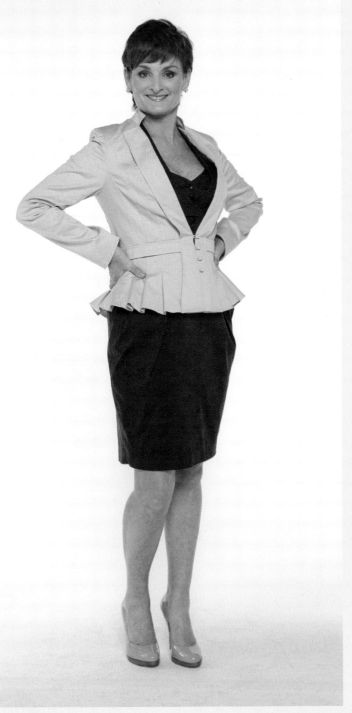

We love this figure-skimming dress and peplum jacket (a jacket that is fitted to the natural waist and kicks out in a little skirt) together. The cream colour is very soft on Deirdre's skin. Team this outfit with an elegant scarf to take you from home to the boardroom.

Add statement jewellery to take you from day to night. A clutch bag and block court shoes will add versatility to this look.

WORK TO PLAY

Shopping (lunch with the girls)

Dresses and coats work really well when you're small, as a single line elongates the body. This structured coat is perfect for Deirdre, as the shoulders and sleeves are narrow, so it doesn't swamp her. Keep the shoulder in line with your body. Over extension can make smaller women look like a mushroom. Wear sleeves as fitted as is comfortable, and to that end, look for Lycra® content in your jackets. The narrower the sleeve, the leaner and more in proportion you will look. These are key details for petites to look for in a coat.

Look for centre panels and vertical detailing – this double-breasted design does the trick. Continue the line with boots rather than shoes. Cropped jackets elongate the legs. Here, we've extended the hemline with an under-hanging skirt in a similar tone.

Our accent is the fabulous red ruffle-front top peeping out from under the coat. Now that would bring a big smile to any girl's face.

The genius nude court shoes further extend Deirdre's legs. They not only look great in summer, but can be worn with pale silver beige tights in the winter, for a very cool look.

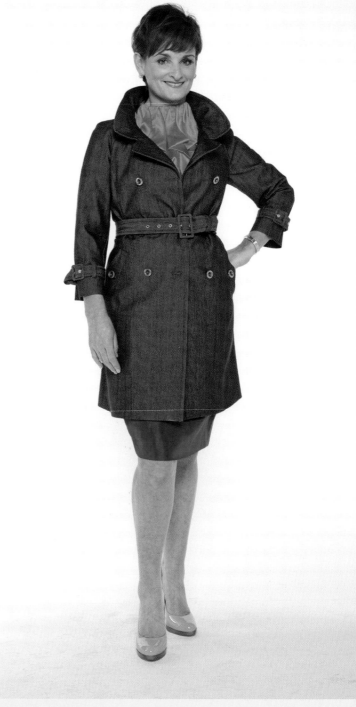

LUNCH WITH THE GIRLS

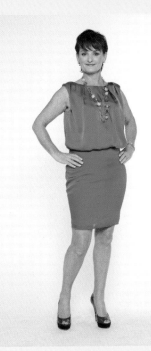

SHE LOOKS AMAZING!
This jade-green dress looks elegant and stunning on Deirdre.

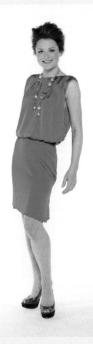

SHE LOOKS AMAZING!
The same dress on Michelle will turn heads.

A petite girl needs some architectural styling to maximise her small frame.

Think deep V-necks (or backs!), defined shoulders, nipped in waists, peplum detail and body-skimming skirt. If you can combine all these elements in one garment, you've found the perfect dress. Think master of the female form, Roland Mouret (google him, you need to know what he does!).

As you know, we also love the idea of injecting colour into your life. This jade-green dress was a fantastic find. Gentle volume on the top half accentuates both Deirdre and Michelle's petite waists and hips giving instant drama. The mismatched shoes, add a humourous edge.

When you begin to master your wardrobe, you can throw in elements of the unexpected. This adds humour and develops your own personal style.

Accessories

- Wedge and platform heels give max. height with min. pain.
- Oversized bags and jewellery can drown a smaller girl.
- Dinky structured bags and small but bold jewellery pieces work better.

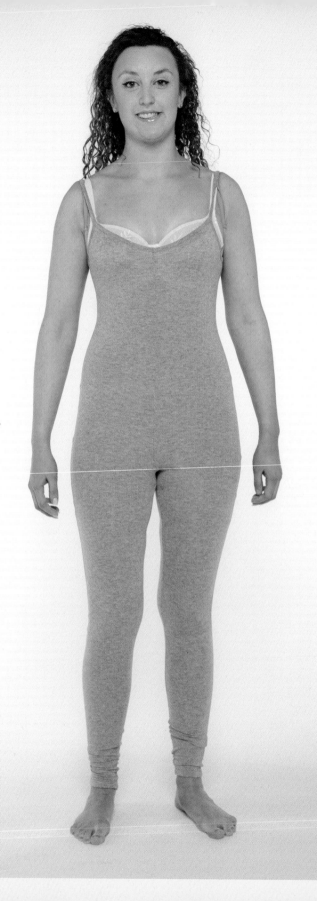

AFTER
STREAMLINED
AMAZONIAN

Shapewear
Nora Gene is wearing a
shapewear body, which
streamlines her mid-section.

AMAZONIAN

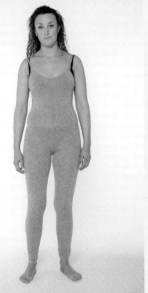

BEFORE

For our ladies with legs that go on forever, here's your style prescription.

Mantra

- Maximise and embrace that height
- Introduce femininity
- Introduce curves
- Break the silhouette with colour and pattern
- Use soft ruffles and chiffons in blouses and tops
- Combine with standard daywear for a feminine edge
- Walk tall, many would like to be standing in your shoes

Avoid

- Manish suiting
- Dark colours head to toe
- Stiff unyielding fabrics

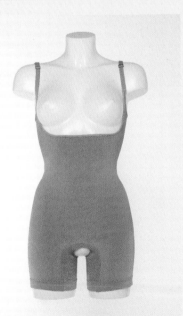

Opposite:
Nora Gene is wearing a shapewear body

Comfort chic (down time)

If you're choosing jeans, go mid or high waist, with a parallel or wide leg. Instead of basic long or short-sleeved tops, try a bit of soft draping. Wrap-around tops and dresses work really well on you. Choose V or scoop necks over high necks. Layer over a feminine camisole to add day-time modesty, interest and depth.

We love the softness of this look on Nora Gene. It's just a top, trousers and cardigan, but it looks so much more. The ruffle neckline is so soft and feminine, and is perfectly complemented by this gorgeous soft navy knit. Incidentally, this cardigan can double as a wrap-over – two for the price of one!

Get yourself a trench coat, which will define your waist and give your casual look an element of structure.

Also worth thinking about, are Capri or three-quarter length trousers. Not everyone can get away with these but you certainly can. Avoid beige and camel tones though, go for navy or grey, and introduce colour on your top half, where it will illuminate your skin and not your hips!

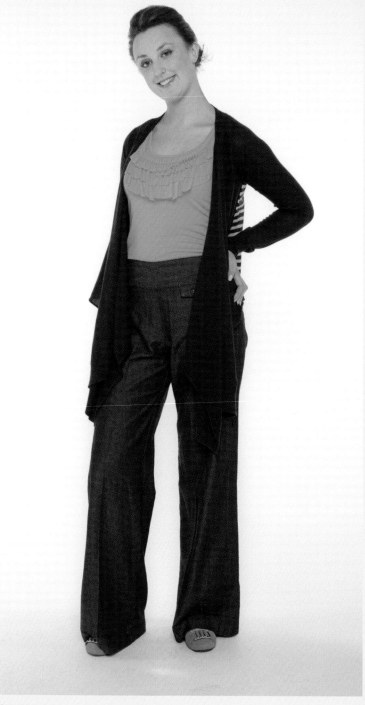

COMFORT CHIC

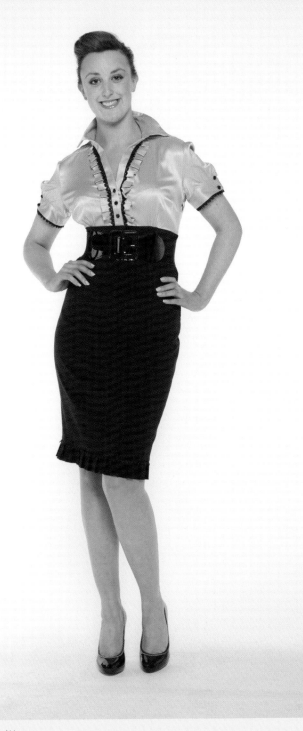

WORK TO PLAY

There are some genius dresses available that give the effect of two pieces combined into one. You all know how we feel about the power of the dress at this stage, and this baby is the ultimate solution for you gorgeous Amazonian babes.

The important thing to remember is to define your silhouette with a break at the waist. That could be a statement belt, or a peplum jacket which is a very flattering waist definer. The key is to introduce softness, without making you feel like an overgrown twelve year old. Femininity doesn't have to be girly, it can smoulder gently, and it certainly does in this classic black and ivory dress.

Our taller girls have one (or should I say two) of the most coveted assets in womankind. Legs up to heaven! Because of this, you have a number of enviable possibilities. Stride purposefully in wide-legged trousers, preferably in a soft crepe (think Katherine Hepburn and Lauren Bacall), or show off those diamond pins in a shorter length skirt. You may not think your legs are great but trust me, 5ft 9" or over, sheer length will get you noticed. They're your legs, learn to love them. We've said it already, but particularly for our taller girls, posture is everything – so walk tall!

We have broken up Nora Gene's silhouette with a graphic yet feminine look. The softness of the dove-grey waistcoat combined with the ivory silk ruffle on the blouse give a feminine slant to what is a strong uncompromising look. This is a perfect example of cleverly introducing feminine elements into a structured combination.

A softly draped wrap dress is also a great asset in every girl's wardrobe. As an enviable Amazonian, you can carry pattern in a way that many can't. Graphic florals are a really nice way to bring grown-up femininity into your wardrobe. A lot of women are flummoxed by scarves, but with your stature, a little billow and flow can look beautiful.

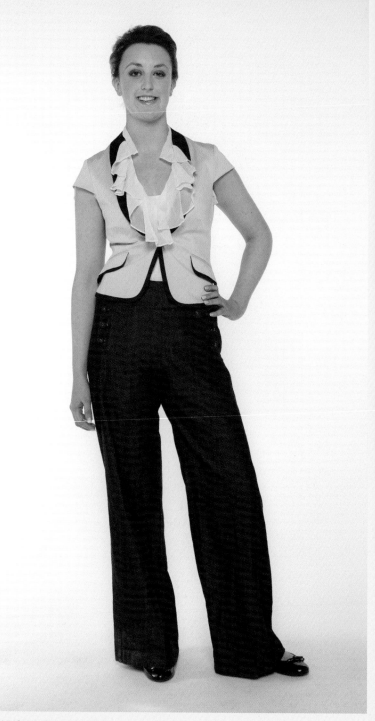

LUNCH WITH THE GIRLS

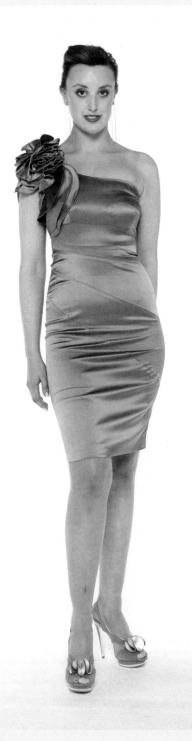

We feel that, when you're tall you carry high drama like many of your smaller sisters can't, so we found Nora Gene this killer number in oyster satin with a shoulder detail that could sashay down any international catwalk.

Tall girls tend to have long torsos, another enviable feature. Use a wide and deep neckline or back-revealing number to maximise that space. A crossover top is a good example. Team with a figure hugging mid-calf pencil skirt, and cinch with a killer belt. Throw caution to the wind and hop into heels; you're tall anyway, so crank it up a notch. If in doubt, kitten heels give elegance without too much elevation, just look at the gorgeous Mrs Obama.

Accessories

- You have the stature to carry off the biggest and boldest accessories.
- Think oversized clutch bags and strong statement jewellery.
- Avoid long beads or long-strapped bags, as they will exaggerate your length.
- Flats look great on you, but don't shy away from heels.
- You are one of the few shapes that can wear an ankle strap.

SHE LOOKS AMAZING!

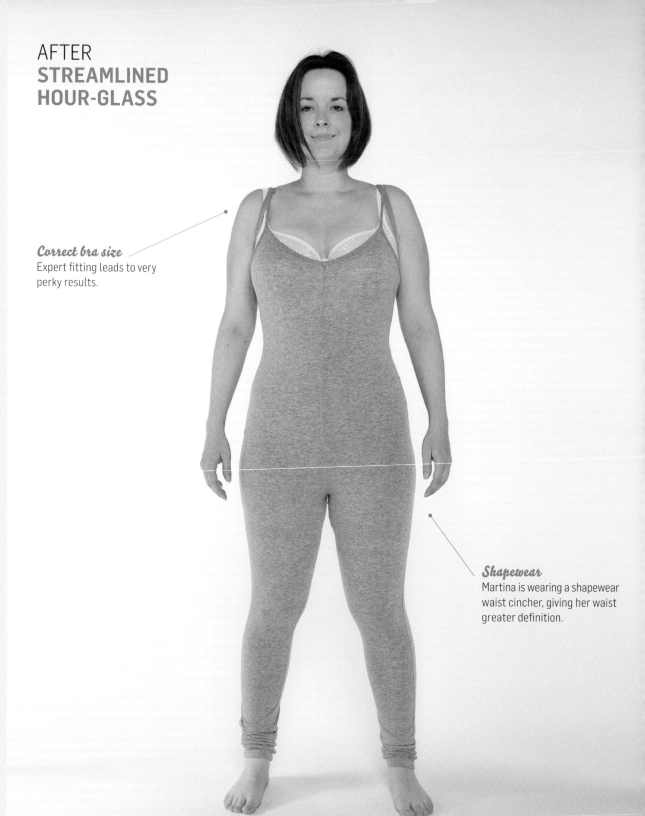

AFTER
STREAMLINED
HOUR-GLASS

Correct bra size
Expert fitting leads to very
perky results.

Shapewear
Martina is wearing a shapewear
waist cincher, giving her waist
greater definition.

HOUR-GLASS

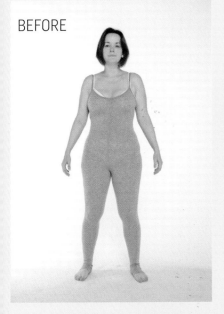

BEFORE

Curvy girls, here are some tips to have you looking like sirens.

Mantra

- I've got curves – and I'm going to use them!
- The most important thing to do with a curvy figure is to define the waist
- Don't apologise for your curves; they've never been hotter
- Go for high-waisted skirts and trousers, it will seem odd at first, but you will soon see the wisdom
- Watch *Some Like It Hot* – it should be your inspiration!

Avoid

- High necklines
- Bold pattern
- A-line shapes
- Baggy tops
- Unstructured and asymmetrical shapes

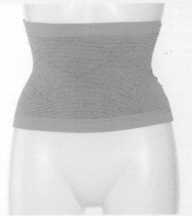

Opposite:
Martina is wearing a shapewear waist cincher

So, it's all about the waist. The addition of a belt to this look lifts it from nice to fabulous. The deep V of the jacket draws the eye down to the narrowest point and the peplum guides the eye down to those sensuous curves. A smart jacket, like this, is such a great investment, because it could literally fit into any of our chosen looks.

These jeans are mid-rise parallels, they make sense of this silhouette, because with curvy girls, what goes out must come back in again.

The soft ivory of the pretty chiffon blouse is so delicate against the skin that it looks barely there, which is why it whispers rather than shouts feminine sex appeal.

A French inspired horizontal striped Breton top can be a very flattering piece. Make sure the neck is boat rather than round. It will slightly exaggerate the line of the shoulder, which in turn makes the waist look smaller. Team with high-waisted jeans or a pencil skirt. Keep the lines simple – let your curves do the talking.

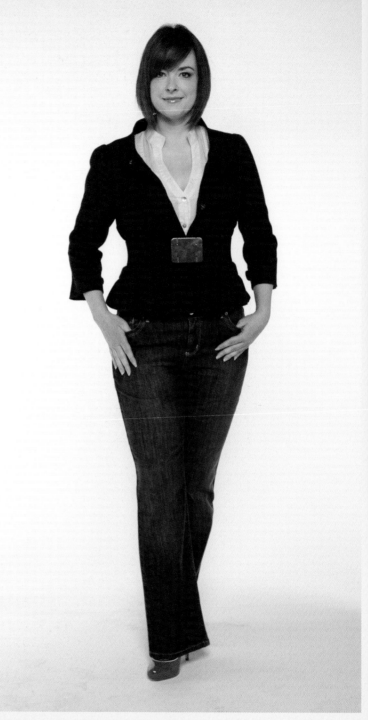

COMFORT CHIC

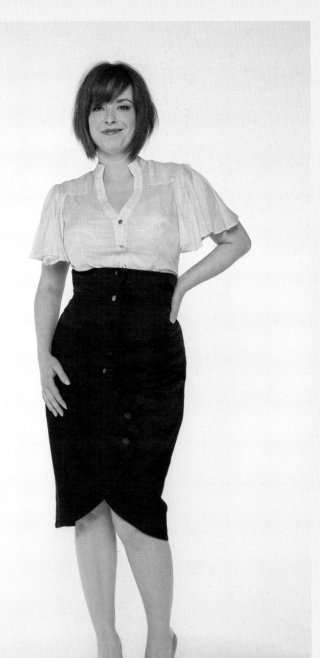

Skirts are much better than trousers on an Hour-glass figure. If you're out of practice, start trying on skirts again, just remember the key is to skim the body contours as much as possible. A pencil skirt that stays close to your silhouette right to its hem is perfect.

This skirt is pure fashion magic and we've used the same chiffon blouse from our comfort chic look. It's so simple, and oh so sexy.

If you are going for trousers, again, high-waists are important; follow the body to the hip and let the line fall into a soft parallel leg. The theory behind this is that trousers that define the inner and outer thigh of a curvy girl can be very unflattering. Keep the lower half dark and bring colour into the top half of your look.

Keep jackets fitted – cropped to the waist works very well.

WORK TO PLAY

Shopping (lunch with the girls)

You know we love dresses, and this subtle mushroom is perfect for daytime chic. The soft wool jersey is pure comfort as it hugs Martina's sensual curves. The clever centre ruffle splits the body in two, making it appear slimmer. We've added a statement belt to spice up the look. A blood-red clutch gives us a colour hit and instant fashion kudos. We know that this dress would be a friend for life, another gentle style statement, to see you through many different occasions.

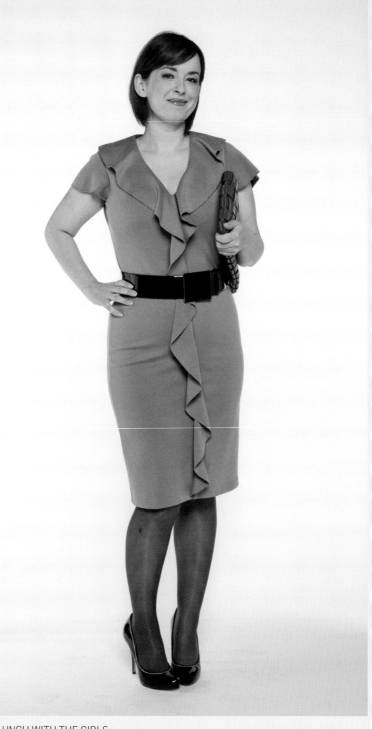

LUNCH WITH THE GIRLS

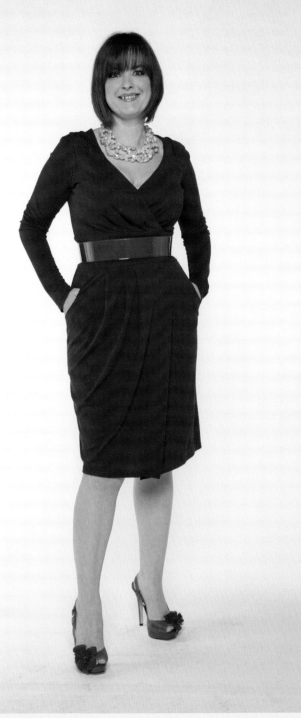

Well we could hardly write a style guide without including a classic wrap dress, could we? Thank you Diane Von Furstenberg for perfecting this art form. The hour-glass can really work this look. Without boobs, the wrap dress is a bit of a damp squib, but as our perfect curvy girl, Martina, shows us, the wrap goes in and out in all the right places. This rich aubergine is a true classic, which we've teamed with tan and purple foot candy. However, hot pink, amber and red accessories would all work really well and give an unexpected and dramatic effect.

Accessories

- Belts, belts, belts.
- Don't be afraid to experiment with colour, using it as a punctuation for your outfit.
- Your natural sexiness screams out for a high heel.
- Classic court shoes are your friends for life, but avoid ankle straps.

SHE LOOKS AMAZING!

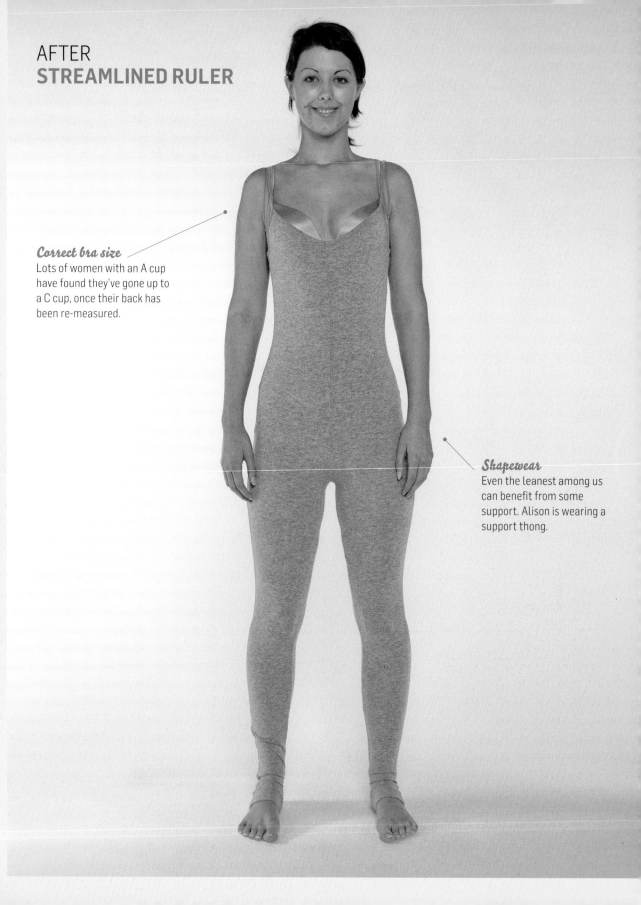

AFTER
STREAMLINED RULER

Correct bra size
Lots of women with an A cup have found they've gone up to a C cup, once their back has been re-measured.

Shapewear
Even the leanest among us can benefit from some support. Alison is wearing a support thong.

RULER

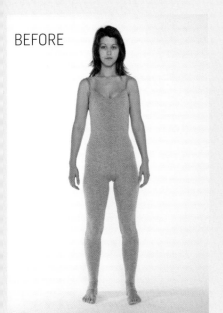

BEFORE

Rulers, your lovely svelte lines are very easily managed. Here are your key tips.

Mantra

- You have model like proportions – rejoice!
- Use every opportunity to create curves and interest
- Turn up the volume in skirts, dresses and shoulders; this will create curves and a waist
- Layering will add depth to any outfit
- Go mad with belts to give you a sexy waist
- Colour blocking will help create a gorgeous silhouette
- Go for bold prints

Avoid

- Garments with no structure
- Anything in a box shape, as it will leave you curveless
- Shapeless baggy clothes will drown your frame
- Dropped waists

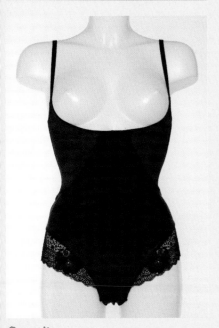

Opposite:
Alison is wearing a shapewear body thong

Comfort chic (down time)

Think gentle flaring on sleeves, skirts and trousers to add definition to your waist and create curves. The central pleat on this top, adds interest and volume and draws Alison's waist in, to make her look much more curvaceous. Wide-leg jeans or trousers fitted on the thigh, will also add dimension to a ruler shape. Try a three-quarter length coat with a fuller skirt, and always belt the waist. Think about using your coat as an accessory to your silhouette. For maximum waist definition, leave the coat open and cinch in the belt at the back. Your lovely long proportions are dramatic and very easy to make more feminine. Think about using strong colours for maximum redefinition.

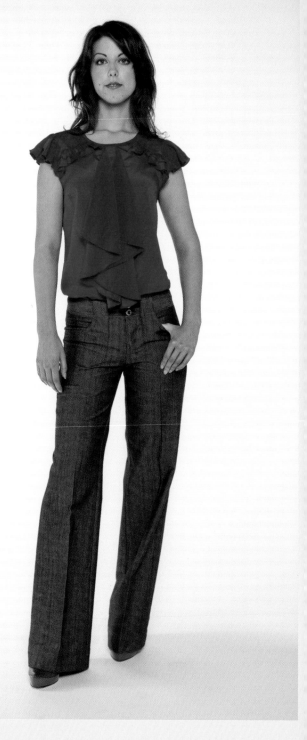

COMFORT CHIC

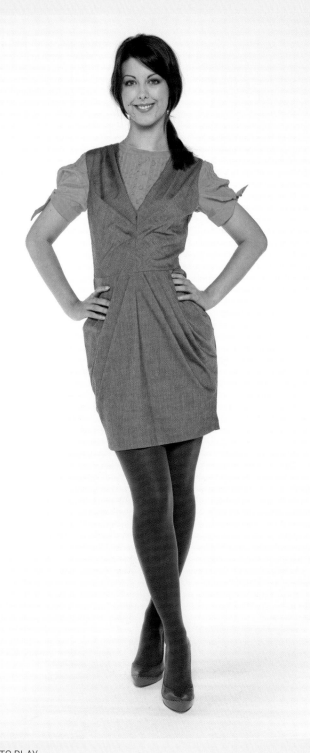

This is the perfect example of clever use of cut and colour. The structured dress with added volume on the hips gives instant femininity. Add the coral blouse with high neck and sleeve detail and Alison has instant va va voom curves. Pop the blouse off and expose those shoulders, for some post-work sex appeal. You are one of the few shapes who could not only wear, but benefit from, a fitted double-breasted jacket (make sure it has the all important shoulder pads). You have created interest in the detail and balance through the cut. Make sure the jacket sits just above the hip, to add shape.

WORK TO PLAY

Shopping (lunch with the girls)

Tulip skirts or anything with volume on the hips, were made with you in mind. With jeans, skirts or dresses go for pockets or embellishment on the hip area to add interest and create those all important curves. Voluminous sleeves bring the eye out at the shoulder, also adding to the magic curve creating effect. When it comes to tops, soft high necklines will help to keep your long torso in proportion. Play with colour and pattern to maximise the affect. You have gorgeous legs, so we advocate showing them off at every given opportunity.

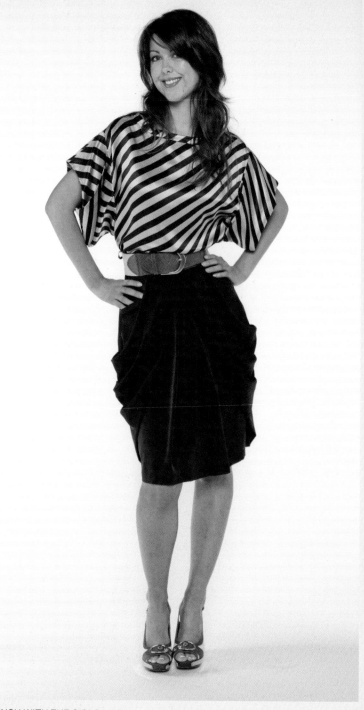

LUNCH WITH THE GIRLS

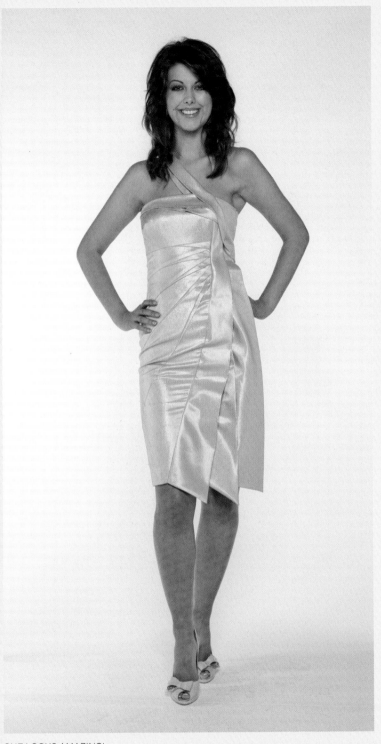

When it comes to dressing you, you lovely model-like Ruler, we want everything to point to your waist and then accentuate your curves, so think sash belts with long tops and voluminous sleeves. A well-cut dress can leave you feeling like a Hollywood starlet. Exposing your shoulders, while wearing the right colour, instantly broadens your top half. Add in a single strap for interest and the mix is perfect. Interesting tailoring, which adds width to your hips, is an absolute smash on you. Add big hair for an Oscar winning look.

Accessories

- Belts, shoulder pads and long statement necklaces, will all help create that waist and curves.
- We love a heel, but you can do kitten and pumps with ease.
- Think big bold jewellery – steer clear of small necklaces and bangles. You are delicate enough.

SHE LOOKS AMAZING!

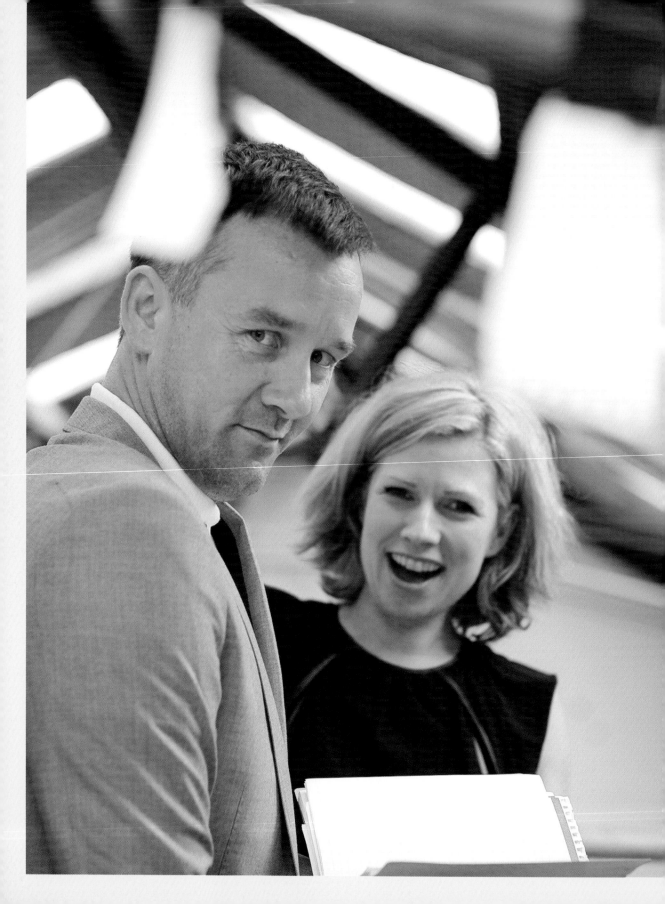

This is a visualisation of our basic principles. We do not advocate that you follow each suggestion to the letter, but rather that you use the theory to draw your own conclusions. Many of you may only have read the section that you believe relates to your own body shape. Just for fun, go back and read the sections for the other shapes. We feel sure that elements of each have something to offer you, even if it's just about learning what's definitely not for you. And remember, getting dressed should be enjoyable. Put the basics in place and the real fun can begin.

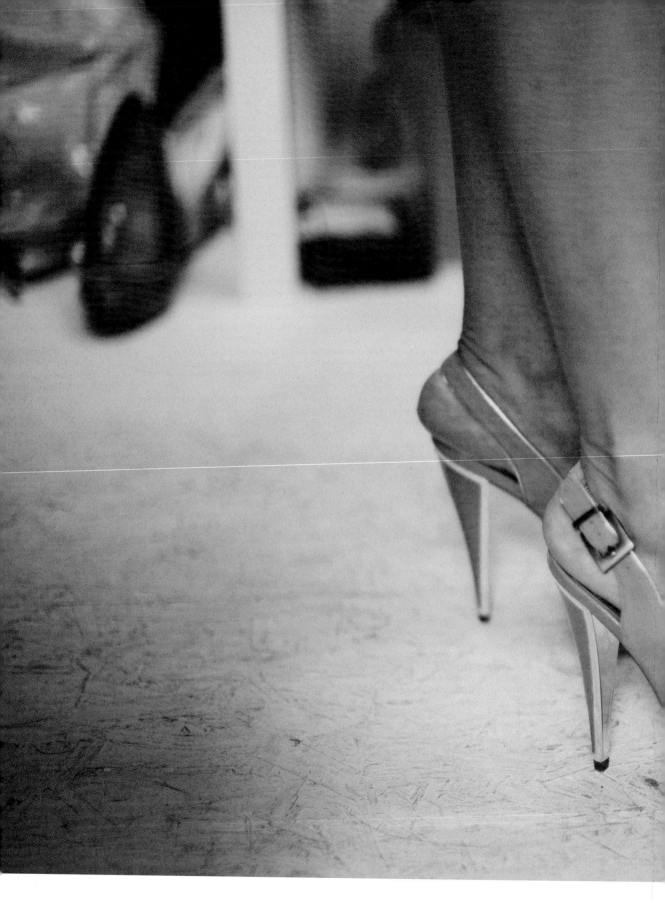

chapter seven

HOW TO ACHIEVE A FULLY FUNCTIONING WARDROBE

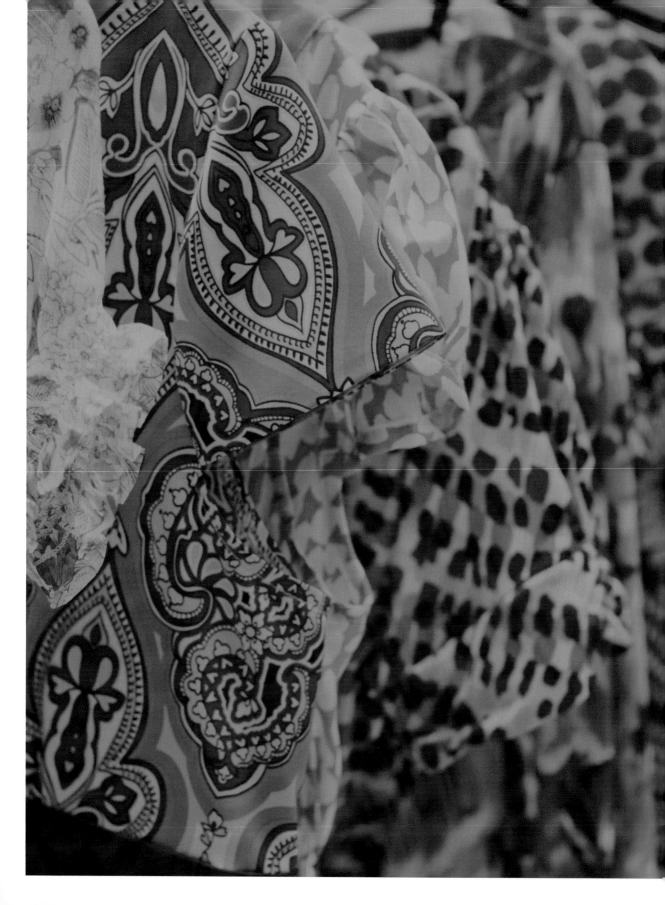

There are essential elements that every woman needs in her arsenal. These are the building blocks of the mystical 'fully functioning wardrobe'. What is a fully functioning wardrobe? Firstly, it can be yours for the taking if you follow our advice. Secondly, it's a collection of pieces that allow you to mix and match, using base elements and accent pieces to fulfil your needs from day to evening, all week long.

The base elements are the work-horses of our wardrobes; items that can be repeatedly used without screaming their presence. They tend to be in neutral colours and classic styles, giving them enduring appeal. For this reason, if we're going to make investments, this is where they should be.

Accent pieces add interest, colour and humour. We all love to know what the latest trends are. Slavishly following them would not be our advice – as we end up as consumerist pawns, rather than the style queens we strive to be. However, it's nice to nod to them and stay current, as accent pieces can give us that edge. The chain stores allow us to buy into new looks, and update our base elements, for a small investment. The quality of our base elements carries the frivolity of our accent pieces, making those inexpensive flourishes look a lot more expensive than they are.

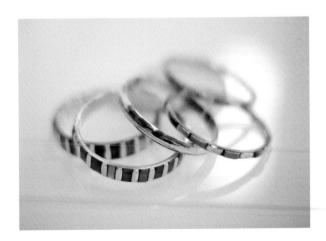

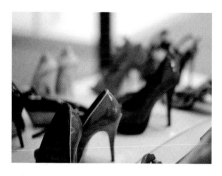

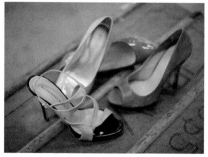

Base elements

TRENCH COAT

A really good trench or light coat, preferably with a belt, is a classic addition to every wardrobe. Don't feel you need to buy this in classic beige. The colour doesn't suit everyone and it isn't the only way to go. If you want to turn a classic piece on its head, go for a bright colour – burnt orange, cornflower blue or even white. If these colours aren't for you, navy is always a good option.

This light coat will be a great friend to you. It's less about the practicality of being warm, and more about being able to give a smart and finished look to a basic outfit. You will feel fully dressed with this flattering garment. Pull the belt to the back and cinch in, to reveal only the centre third of your body. Then people will not register the bits that they can't see – instant body sculpting!

SUNGLASSES

We never go anywhere without sunglasses. Spend time finding a shape that suits your face.

The glamour quotient is directly related to size, so as they say: 'Go Large'. They don't have to be expensive, as ever, the high street stores are doing great versions of the heavy hitters.

SMART TROUSERS

A smart pair of trousers is a great basic. Three classic styles that are great to own are straight leg, parallel leg and wide leg. Trousers can be difficult to get right, particularly if you have curves. Spend time finding the right ones and look for Lycra® content for comfort. Many of us find that what fits on the hip and thigh doesn't fit on the waist. Don't be disheartened, if they're right in every other way then have them tailored to fit, there's no shame in it.

SMART JEANS

A lot of us have misconceptions about denim and consider it to be sloppy casual wear. Not any more. Smart cut denim, in indigo dye, is a great building block for a modern stylish wardrobe. See our tips in chapter 6 to choose the right fit for you.

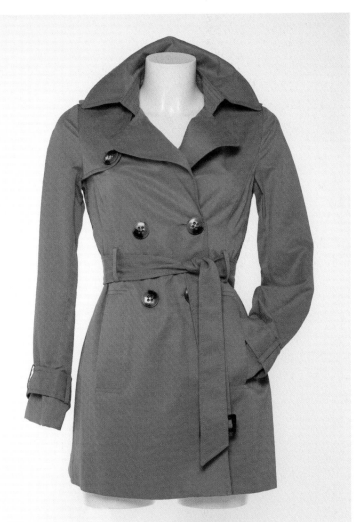

Classic straight legged trousers

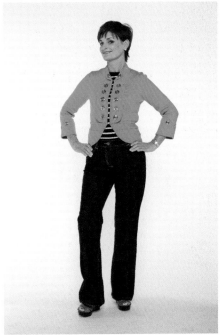

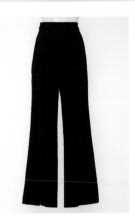

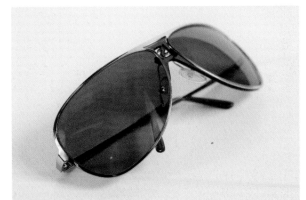

Sunglasses – the bigger the better

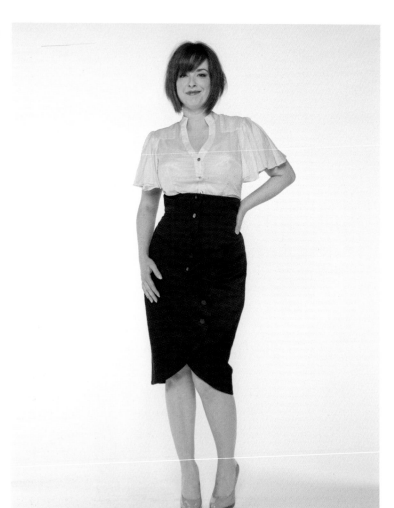

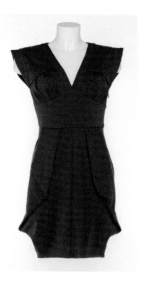

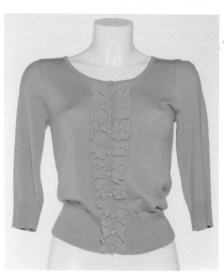

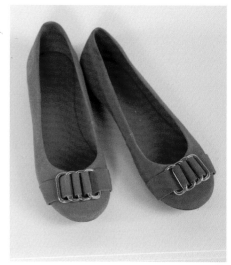

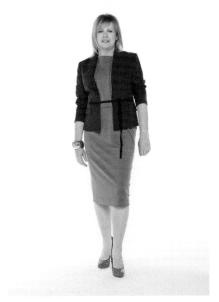

An outfit that will take you from day to night

DAY TO NIGHT DRESS/ POWER SHIFT

This is the basic piece for every style queen. Get this right and the price per wear index will fall to nothing! (Haven't heard of it? Divide the price of a garment by the number of times that you will wear it and you have its 'price per wear!') So many of these lists say every woman needs a little black dress (LBD). We disagree, it can be black but it doesn't have to be. Try navy, you will be pleasantly surprised. Keep it simple, to ensure enduring value and usage. Remember that this item can have multiple personalities, depending on how you accessorise.

PENCIL SKIRT

You must, must, must own one of these. Again, don't feel you have to go for black. If you have the nerve, or are top heavy, try oatmeal tones; if not try navy, brown or grey, these are much softer alternatives to the demon black.

SHORT FITTED JACKET

A short jacket, for instance one to the waist, can have an incredible figure-defining effect. Your choice of style is, of course, your own – blazer, military or even mini trench. Just make sure that you're not introducing too much volume, this item's job is to streamline the silhouette.

CASHMERE JUMPER

Anyone who has never experienced cashmere is missing out on one of life's simplest pleasures. It used to be the preserve of the rich but, again, thanks to the high street chains, it is now completely accessible. We love a slouchy style with a V-neck in a soft tone. You will feel comforted when you wear it. It's a sartorial hug. Team with smart jeans and pumps, or wrap yourself up on the couch – such is the joy of wearing cashmere.

FLAT PUMPS

We're the world's greatest high heel fans. But even we recommend the addition of flat leather pumps to your wardrobe. Team with your 'day to night dress' or cropped trousers and your cashmere V-neck (don't forget those sunglasses!), and imagine yourself as Jackie O!

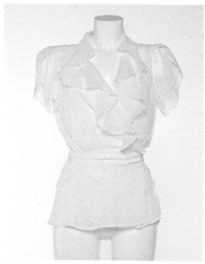

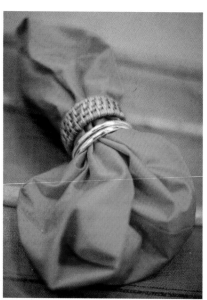

SHEER BLOUSE

The blouse has made an incredible comeback, and not without good cause. As far back as the Victorians, an embellished blouse gave silhouette and femininity in equal measure. The 1970s saw small screen icons, like Mary Tyler Moore and Candice Bergen, master the art of a good blouse. Now Kate Moss shows us how it's done. Go sheer and layer with delicate camisoles to give a wonderfully sexy yet demure look.

Accent pieces

STATEMENT JEWELLERY

Some of the most stylish people we know wear the largest and most dramatic jewellery, and we're not talking diamonds. Accessorising can be daunting, but once you've got the basics in place, it is the icing on the cake.

Accent colours

Colour has an amazing and instantaneous effect on your mood. Certain colours have their moment from season to season. From exotic sallow complexions to the palest beauty, everyone has an accent colour to suit them. Don't be tempted to buy into a colour just because the fashion police tell you 'it's all in'. However, if the colour of the season suits you, go for it, and you will find that it will have longevity in your collection.

Pattern

Pattern and print can be very fashion fickle, with some notable exceptions, such as Pucci and Missoni. These labels are serious investments with proven endurance. However, pattern can be a great way to channel the look of a season, be it animal, geometric or floral.

Accessories

Tiny subtleties in style keep us spending our hard earned cash. Accessories are the easiest way to look current and stylish. They are also a lot cheaper than buying a whole new wardrobe (unless you have a Carrie Bradshaw-like addiction!). Coloured shoes are among the

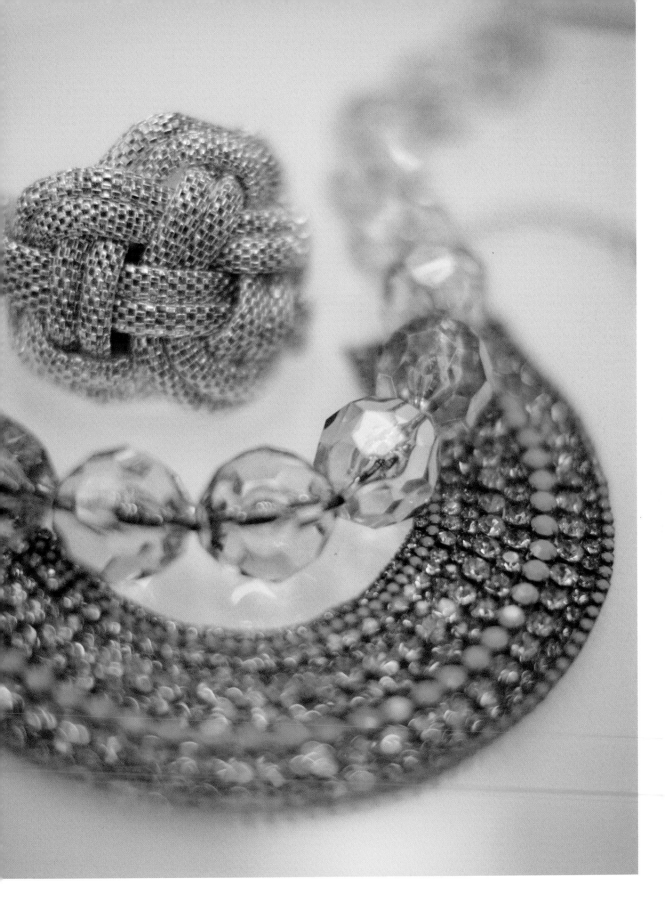

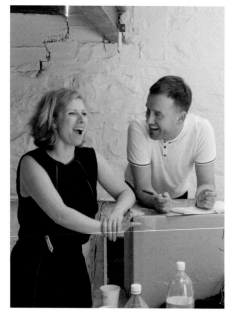

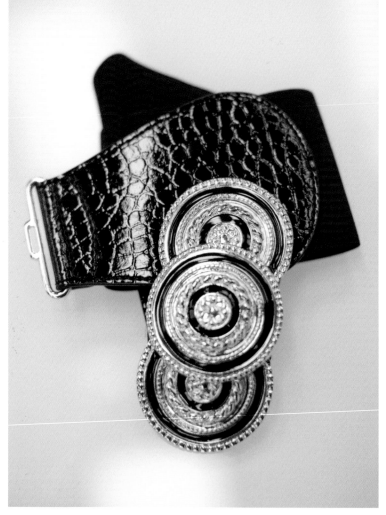

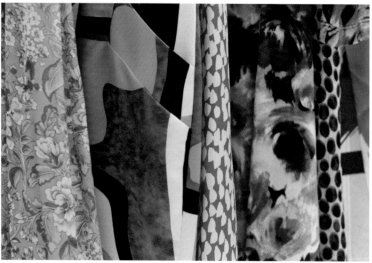

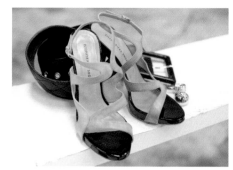

most fun things to buy. Even if you're not spending a fortune on them, there's something fabulously decadent about hot-pink or lizard-green shoes.

The days of matching shoes and bag are over. Somehow, it always looks a bit 'Mother of the Bride'. In the same way, while jewellery sets are charming, they often have more cachet when worn separately.

Accessories are a great way to personalise your wardrobe. Don't forget about hats and gloves, and we don't mean bobble hats and mittens! Hats for daywear can look striking, and there are beautiful wearable versions available. If you've invested in a classic coat in a dark neutral, pump up the fun with some bold coloured leather gloves.

We believe that getting dressed each morning should be pain free and enjoyable. When you master a fully functioning wardrobe, on your worst days, your wardrobe will offer reliable old friends to get you out the door, on your best days you will feel vital and sexy. One thing is for sure – you will never again look into your wardrobe and say, 'I've nothing to wear!'

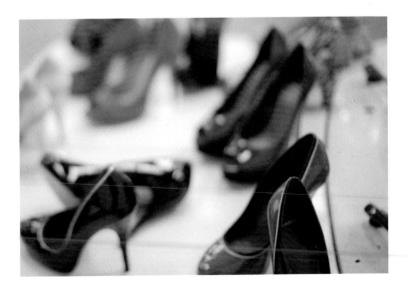

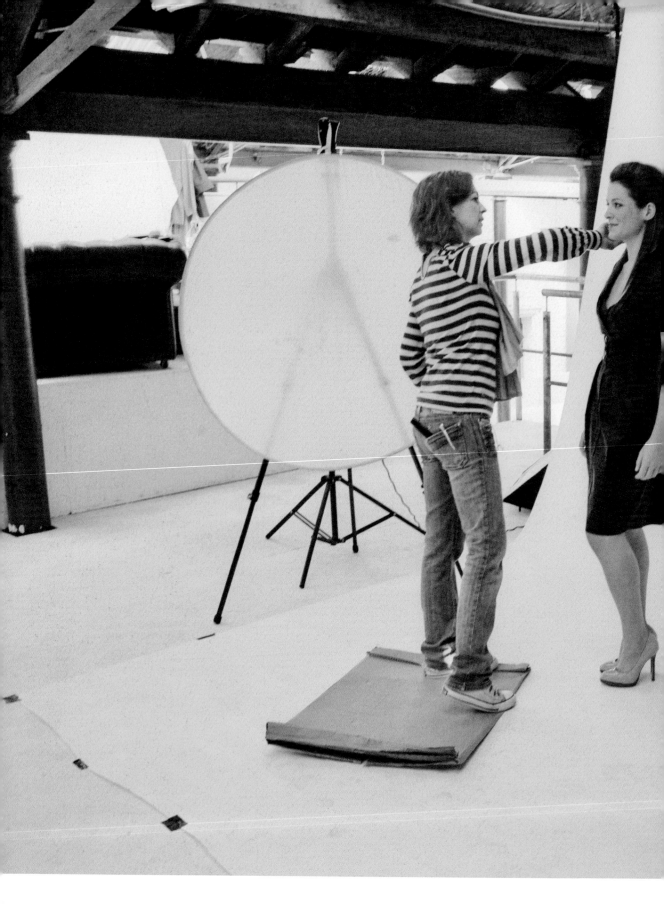

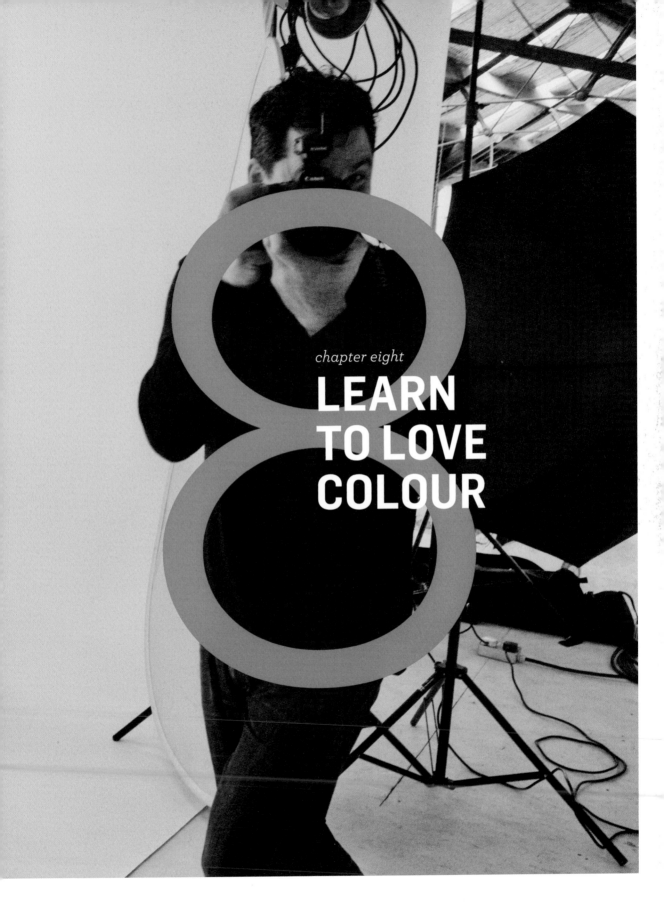

chapter eight

LEARN
TO LOVE
COLOUR

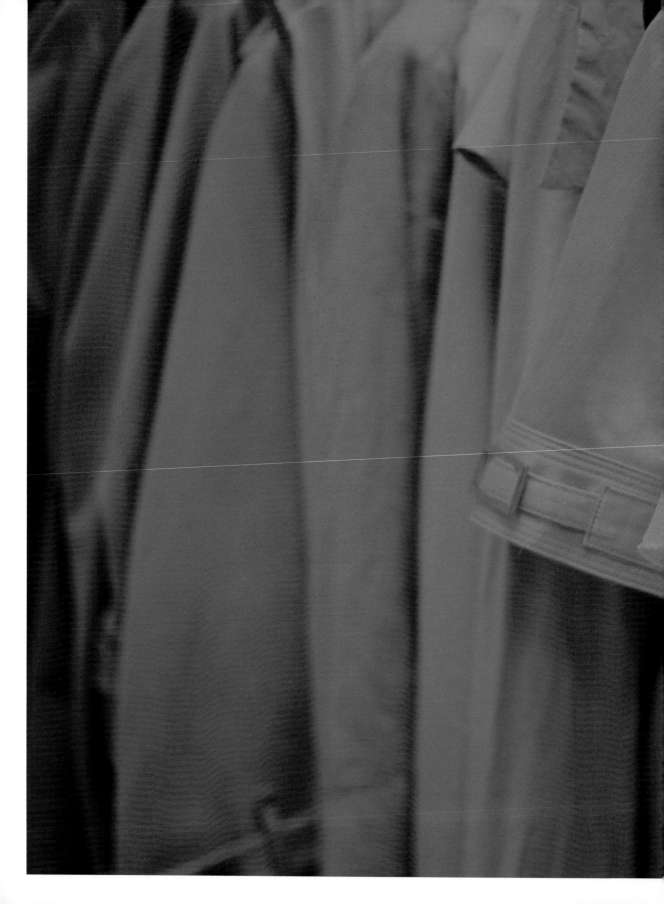

How to build a new colour palette

Diana Vreeland famously said: 'Pink is the navy blue of India'. Unfortunately, for many of us, black is the navy blue of modern life.

Many of you have told us that you have a psychological problem with wearing colour.

And we cannot believe the number of you who cover your fabulousness in a protective shroud of black. Now, don't get us wrong, black has a very valid place in every woman's wardrobe. Where would we be without the iconic images of Audrey Hepburn in *Breakfast at Tiffany's*, showing us all how it's done? The problem occurs when black ceases to be a punctuation mark, and begins to be a default mechanism.

We've spoken about how to tackle the architecture of your wardrobe, now we need to focus on the palette.

As with everything we have discussed, we urge you to really think about the colours in your wardrobe, and have a grand plan.

For simplicity, we've broken the palette down into two categories – neutrals and accents.

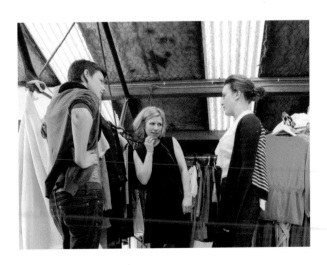

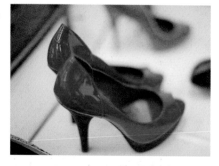

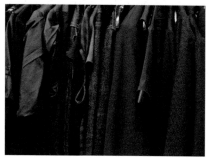

Neutrals

DARK NEUTRALS

As we've already discussed, every wardrobe needs base elements as the building blocks of style.

Imagine yourself on a mission to find the perfect pair of smart trousers or pencil skirt.

What colour is in your head? We're guessing it's black. But black is not necessarily the best base colour for your wardrobe. On a day-to-day basis, it can be harsh on our delicate skin tones, and far from elevating for our moods.

With a little bit of effort we can step away from our reliance on the dark force and into the softer world of what we call 'dark neutrals'. Dark neutrals are the varied tonal world of brown, navy and grey. The next time that you're in a clothing store, try the following exercise. Instead of reaching for a jacket, coat or trousers in black, see if they've got it in one of the dark neutrals.

Navy is a friendly colour for pretty much every skin tone. Brown tones are great on dark haired beauties, but greys are best avoided, as they can bring out grey tones in a dark complexion. Lucky blondes can wear it all. The trick is to find out which of these colours work for you.

Strangely, or maybe not, the best way to dip your toe into this world is with footwear. It's very hard to make dark neutrals work if all your shoes are black. In recent years the wonderful chain stores expanded the colour range of their basic footwear. If you want to invest in winter boots in navy, grey or brown – no problem!

You will be amazed at the softness that you can achieve with no loss of practicality. Even for those of you unsure of colour, this should not be too big a stretch. Remember that there is only one black, but buying into dark neutrals gives you a huge tonal range from which to choose.

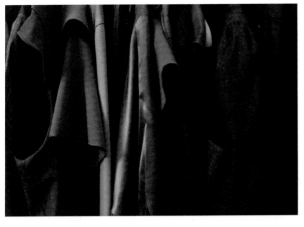

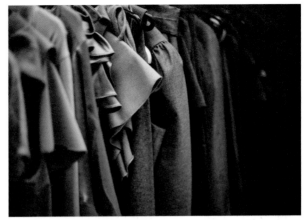

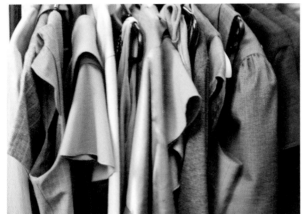

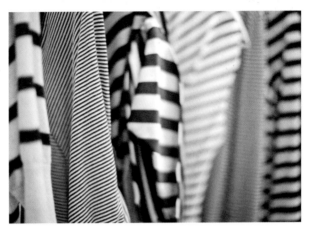

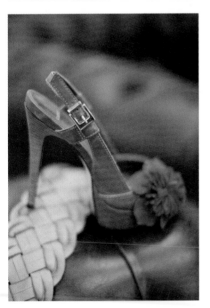

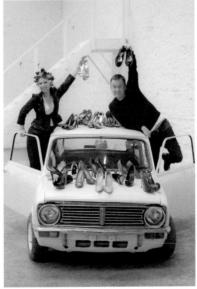

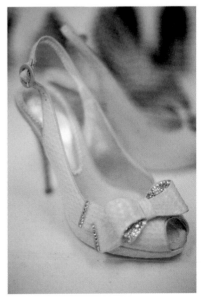

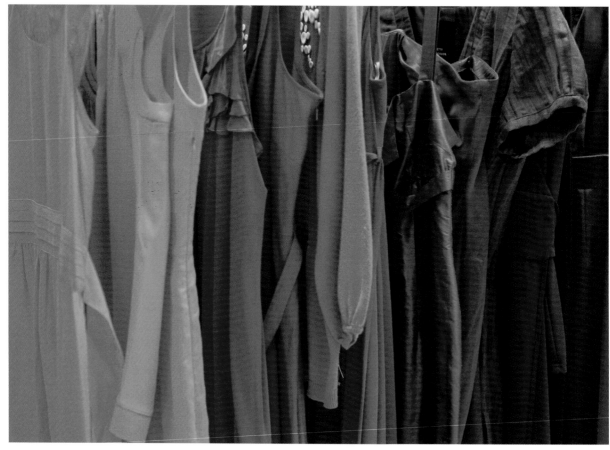

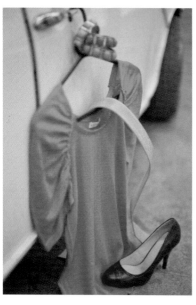

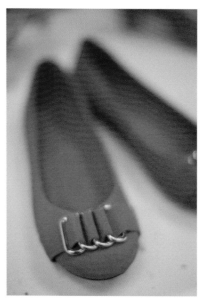

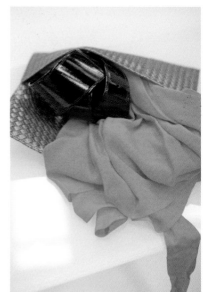

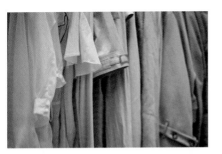

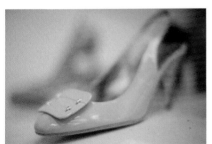

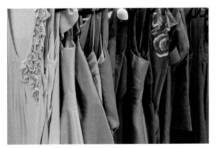

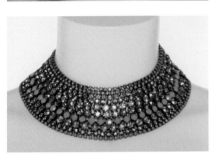

Traditionally, the standard office uniform was black tailoring with a white shirt or blouse. When executed well this look can be sharp and sassy. However, because it becomes the path of least resistance for armies of working women, it's hard to get excited about its impact. It is very easy to inject softness and femininity into work-wear without losing your professional and chic image.

When approaching that rail, fight the instinct driving you directly to the white blouse, think about replacing it with a softer tone of ivory, oyster or dove grey. Coupled with your newly discovered dark neutrals, you will see a beautiful richness emerging that is impossible to achieve with black and white.

Accents

COLOUR

Deep, rich, tonal softness is now yours. This is a great starting point for your wardrobe and chosen carefully, these pieces will become reliable old friends, to be mixed and matched, taking you from the supermarket to the boardroom.

But you're not finished yet! To personalise your style and get you genuinely excited about your wardrobe and your image, we need some emphasis. This can be achieved with accent colours. Because so many of you have told us that you're colour phobic, we suggest that you introduce this incredible mood enhancer gently, through accessories. Shoes, scarves, bags and jewellery can represent the beginning of an affair with the colours that you will grow to love.

Our favourite palette for depth and vibrancy is what we called 'jewel tones' – amethyst purple, emerald green, sapphire blue, amber and ruby red. Even the names draw you in. These are naturally occurring colours, and that might be the key to their success. Once you get hooked, there will be no going back.

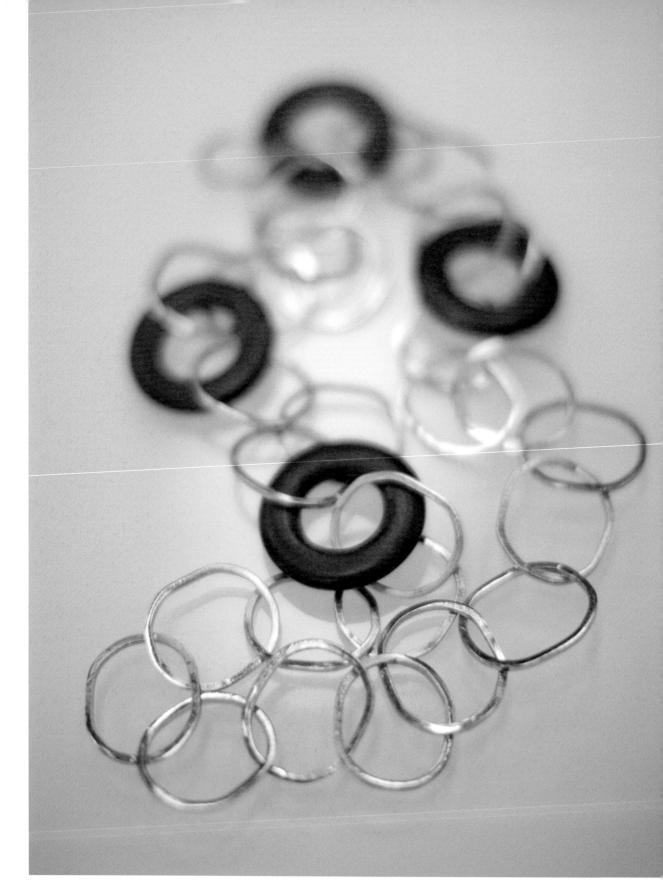

Every woman we have worked with has been amazed by the power of colour – you will immediately feel and look brighter. Don't just stick to our colour suggestions, start finding out for yourself which colours work for you. With your dark and light neutrals as a safety net, you can start to build up your courage. You might even become adept at the art of colour blocking. This is mixing strong colours together, a green top with a purple skirt, or a pink top with deep red trousers. This may sound crazy, and it is difficult to pull off, but it can work wonderfully.

PATTERN

We consider pattern to be advanced colour. Some people love it; others avoid it like the plague. It can be tricky to get right, and is a vast and complex world, from delicate florals to jungle prints. Think about the effect that a print will have on your silhouette. A big bold pattern will engulf our Petite ladies. Our Amazonians and Rulers should avoid long linear patterns, so they need to be chosen carefully. Use pattern to draw the eye to your assets and away from the bits of yourself that you wish to conceal. To that end, pattern is often better chosen in separate pieces rather than dresses or two-pieces. All of this is entirely dependent on the pattern, so make sure you try on and proceed with caution.

The colour palette is an often overlooked element of our wardrobe. While we might have an exacting colour plan for our living rooms, we often haven't thought about where we want to go with our clothes. Preparation is everything, follow the guidelines in this chapter and you will be rewarded with a collection that not only makes you look gorgeous, but that also lifts your spirits.

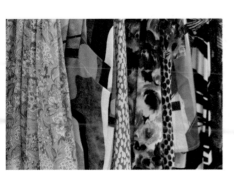
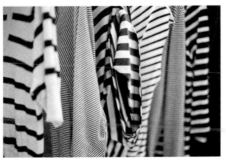

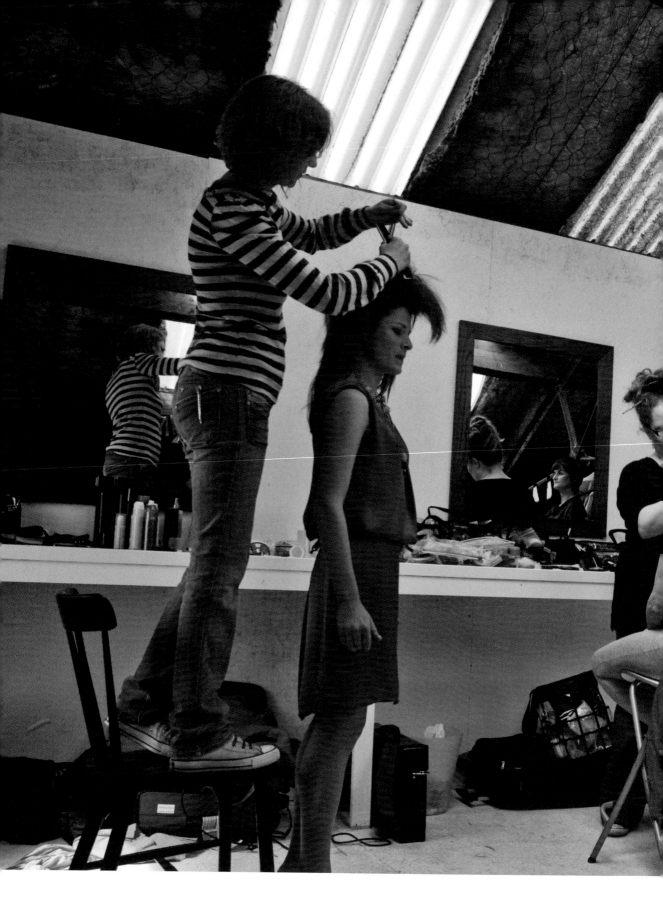

chapter nine
HOW TO SHOP

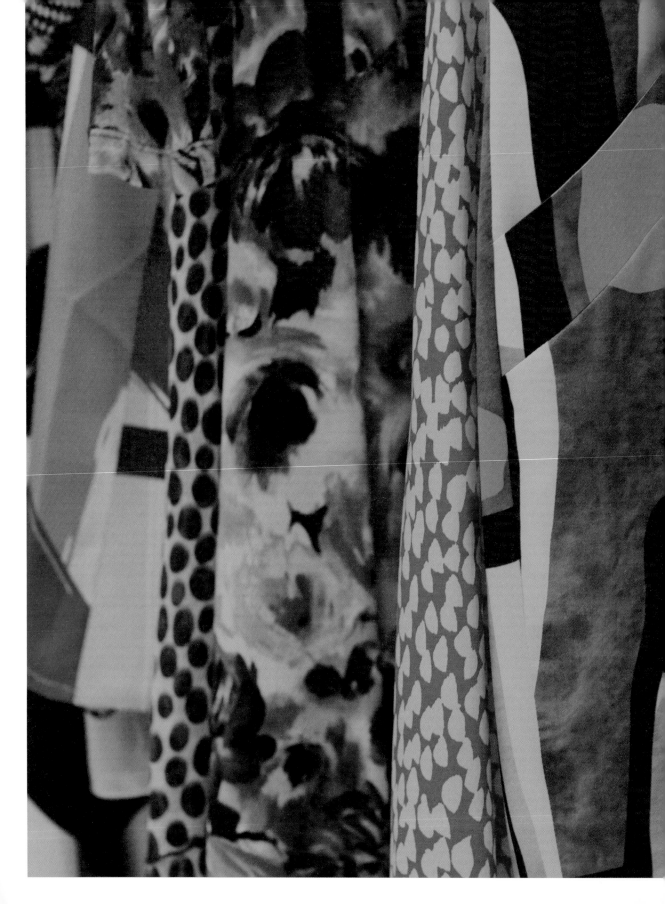

We have helped many women, both on and off the show, to successfully transform their look. One of the things that has become abundantly clear to us is that, contrary to popular belief, most of you hate shopping. We know clothes, and we know how to shop, and we are here to show you how to take the pain away and become knowledgeable, confident and stylish shoppers.

Shopping is not about amassing a monster collection of all the latest must-haves. Rather, it is about being the architect of your own wardrobe. We will show you how to develop a grand plan for your own personal style, embellishing it with flourishes of fun along the way.

The days of randomly buying for a quick adrenalin hit are gone, and frankly, good riddance! This book is about arming you with the knowledge that you need to create a fully functioning wardrobe with a healthy lifespan. That means having a plan!

Preparation is everything, and that's why we've asked you to follow the rigorous and, sometimes, difficult steps in this book. We've asked you to take a cold hard look at your body shape, and identify what you dislike and what you can love about what you see in the mirror. We've asked you to get fitted for the correct size bra. If you have done that you will already see an amazing difference. Add some controlling shapewear, and your contours will be altogether more appealing. We've asked you to enlist a trusted friend to become your style buddy: a warm-hearted confidant with whom you can find mutual and positive support.

If you have followed these steps, then you are ready to shop.

In chapter 1 we detailed a three-day pre-shopping plan. This is very important, even if you have decided to fly solo. Having followed those steps, you will now have a plan for what you need in your wardrobe. This should include a colour palette (see chapter 8) and a list of looks that work for you. Also, you should have a clear sense of what your wardrobe needs to provide for you.

How to read a store

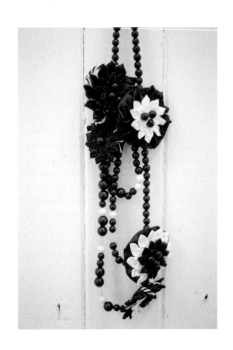

Many of you have told us that you just don't understand the message that shops are trying to communicate. When you get inside the front door, all you see is a mass of clothes in a variety of colours. This can cause utter confusion.

Retailers use merchandising to communicate with their customers. All shops are merchandised into sections; if you learn this you can begin to tackle each shop bit by bit, instead of being overwhelmed.

Firstly, bring to mind your grand plan. Why are you in the shop? Look at the first block of clothes and identify the story they are telling. Is it work wear, casual wear, high fashion or occasion wear?

Generally, stores will entice you in with their most appealing displays, just inside the door. Most of us are magpies at heart, attracted by bright colours and a little bit of bling. You will often find that a few key bright or sparkly items give a strong identity to what are essentially basic pieces, cleverly put together. The important thing here is to take your time. Rushing around in a panic leads to impulse buys and bad choices.

If you see something that appeals to you, don't go running straight to the fitting room. Put it under your arm and work the rest of the store, before committing to taking your clothes off. Pull two sizes, the size that you think you are, and a size bigger. When you try on, try the

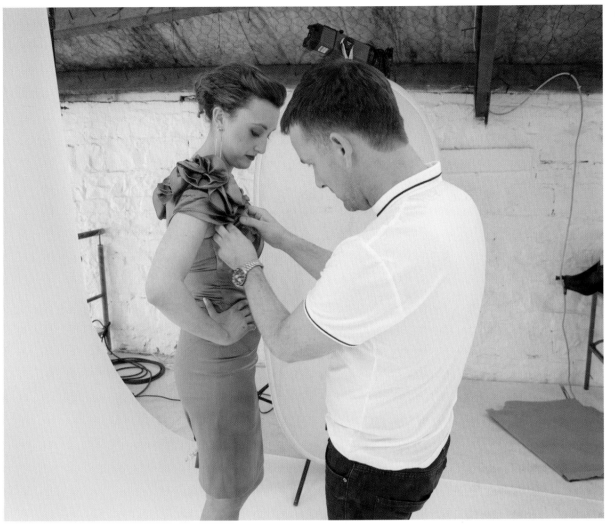

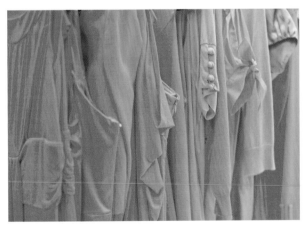

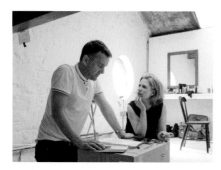

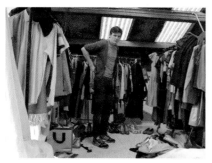

bigger one first. If it fits, then you've saved yourself the embarrassment of calling the indifferent shop assistant to get you the next size up. If it's too big, you have the smaller one to try. If that's too big, take delight in waving through the curtain and asking for the next size down.

Sizing

It's important, at this stage, to discuss the strange and often cruel world of sizing. Our opinion is that it means little or nothing. There is no universal scale and never will be. Sizing depends on who designed the garment, where they are from, where the garment was manufactured and, importantly, how much it costs.

Continue to work your way through the shop, section by section. Pull styles and sizes with abandon. If something appeals to you on any level, pull it. The time that it takes you to cover the whole shop, gives your brain the space it needs to process some of your choices.

When you've done the full circuit, find room on a rail and hang what you've got. You will probably look at half of it and ask, 'What was I thinking?' That's okay, it's better to enter into this with a spirit of bravery rather than fearfulness.

Note: A German 14 is very different to an Italian 14, and very, very different to an American 14. Enlightened retailers see the benefit of generous sizing, however, the margins for cheaper garments are so tight that every centimetre counts, and often fabric is scrimped on to cut costs.

FEAR OF TRYING ON

There's a lot of fear wrapped up in the practice of clothes shopping. You've told us that you're intimidated by the shop itself and by its staff. You've also told us that you'd rather do endless chores than strip off and get changed 'in public'. Well, we're sorry but only by trying clothes on, can you truly understand your own body and the clothes themselves.

The more clothes you try on, the more knowledgeable you will become. The number of women who we've met who have wardrobes full of still tagged garments is frightening.

In the main, this is a result of not trying on in the shop. We all have good intentions of returning unwanted items, but life has a habit of getting in the way of our best intentions. So, try on in the shop. This will not only give you the power to know what really suits you – it will save you hard-earned money!

When you're trying on clothes, it's important to have the right footwear. Either bring your own with you, or ask the shop assistant for a pair in your size that will complement what you are about to try on. Don't be afraid to ask for what you need. Remember, you are the customer; the sales team is there to assist you.

When you've tried your selection, you will probably experience an impulse reaction: 'I love it', 'I hate it' or 'I'm not sure'. Obviously, 'I hate it' is easy to deal with – get rid of it.

IF YOUR FIRST REACTION WAS LOVE, ASK YOURSELF A FEW QUESTIONS:

- Do I love it because I already own it in a slightly different form?
- Do I love it because it's hiding my bad bits or because it's accentuating my assets?
- Do I love it because it looks great on someone else or because it looks great on me?

If you're satisfied with your answers to those questions, here are some more:

- Will I wear this garment?
- What can I wear over or under it?
- Does it make my wardrobe more useable?

If you're still happy, congratulations, you've struck gold!

As you become more proficient at shopping, you will begin to realise which shops work for you. The benefit of this is that, generally, within one store, sizes tend to remain constant. Also, as you shop there, try to recognise faces from your previous visit and see if you can make yourself known to the staff. Do this gently – you don't want them to think that you're looking for a new best friend, merely for some attentive service.

Know your rights

There are two basic reasons why we return goods. Firstly, because there was something technically wrong with it, and secondly, because we are human, and we changed our mind due to aesthetics or fit. Let's deal with the technical stuff first, more on bad decisions later.

If a purchase is faulty, your rights are clearly laid out by law. As a consumer you have basic entitlements. Your unspoken contract with the retailer demands that the goods you purchase are of 'satisfactory quality'. This is a legal term, which protects you against goods being damaged or faulty or unable to withstand normal wear and tear.

The item must be 'fit for its purpose', another bit of legalese, which means that you are entitled to expect the item to perform the task for which it was designed. Whereas you would not expect to run a marathon in a pair of stilettos, you could justifiably assume that a pair of running shoes would last the course. If they don't, boomerang them!

Your final weapon in consumer law is that your purchase should be 'as described'. This is perhaps the vaguest area. If, under the soft lighting and music of your favourite store, a shop assistant told you that the frock you were trying on was navy, and you took it home to find out that it was black (and you know how we feel about black!), you are within your rights to return the item on the basis that it was not 'as described'.

If you are dissatisfied with your purchase, for any of the above reasons, you can exercise your 'right to reject', that is, to return it.

So, these are your rights and the retailer has rights too.

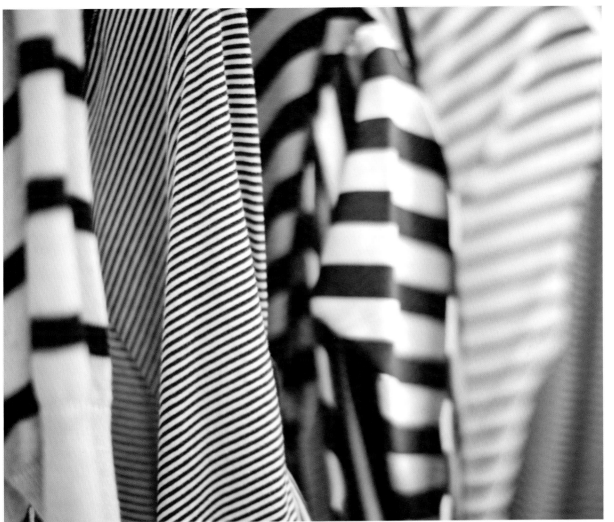

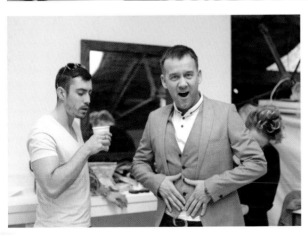

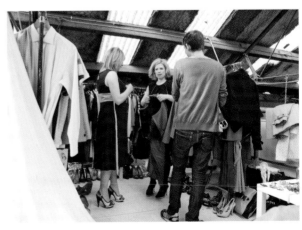

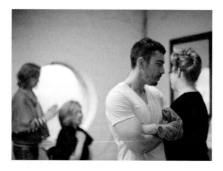

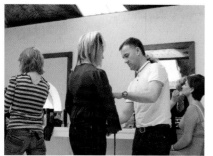

When you return faulty goods, it is within the retailer's right to offer you one of three things. These are called 'the three Rs': repair, replacement or refund. Now, let's be clear about this, contrary to what you might think, a retailer is within their rights to start the ball rolling with repair. This may not please you, but as it's at the discretion of the management, dancing up and down and keening is no guarantee of satisfaction.

Keep your head, and allow due process. When the repair is complete, it is up to you to decide whether you are satisfied with the results. In other words, has the repair permanently returned the goods to perfect condition. If not, we move on to the next step.

The management can now offer you a replacement or refund. Given that you've already been through the wringer, brace yourself; chances are they'll plump for replacement.

If they cannot replace the item with an exact replica, finally, you are entitled to a refund.

You'd think that the matter ends there – it doesn't. The manner of your refund is at the discretion of, you've guessed it, the retailer. You can be offered cash, credit card refund or cheque. Take what you're offered – you've just won the battle.

It is illegal to have a sign stating: 'No refunds' or 'No refunds on sale items', unless it is accompanied by the disclaimer: 'this does not effect your statutory rights'. What this actually means is that the retailer will not offer you the opportunity to change your mind for purely aesthetic reasons. In the case of faulty goods, all your entitlements apply.

Now we get to the second scenario you've changed your mind. You thought you liked it in the shop, but brought it home and realised that it was a cruel and hideous mistake. In this instance, we're afraid that you are at the mercy of the retailer.

Luckily, most fashion stores appreciate the benefit of good customer relations. Take note of the 'window of return'. Every retailer who offers this service has a cap on the period of time within which you must return your unwanted purchase. This ranges from seven days to three generous months – most apply a 14 day return rule. If you return after this period, you are, once again, dealing with the discretion of the retailer.

HOW TO RETURN AN UNWANTED ITEM

If you are returning something that you bought in error, remember, the error was yours. Even if the sales assistant told you that you reminded her of Angelina Jolie in that dress, the term *caveat emptor* comes into play. 'Buyer beware' means that, as with all things in this life, you have to keep your wits about you.

When returning to the shop, try to have a calm and pleasant disposition. You are much more likely to get what you want with charm than with indignance and fury.

Always remember that sales assistants have seen it all, including unscrupulous divas who buy an item, wear it and return it as new for a refund. Any shop assistant worth their salt will sniff that one out.

Shopping should be fun. Relax into it, take your time and when you've struck gold and are in a position to purchase – do it. There is nothing worse than having to panic buy for an occasion: follow our advice and your wardrobe should be able to provide stunning outfits for all occasions. At most, some clever accessory shopping should be all that's required.

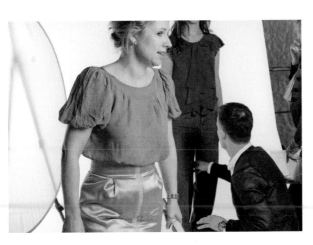
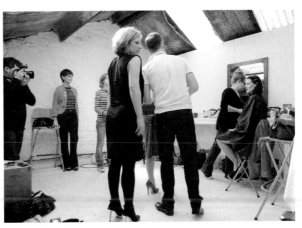

Where to shop

Now that you are equipped to navigate your way around the shops and aware of your consumer rights, it's time to go shopping.

There is an ever-growing choice of clothing retailers with lots to offer – everything from timeless classics to outrageous accessories. In this chapter we divide the clothing retailers into categories, and look at what each category does well. Regardless of budget, value for money is high on everyone's agenda. For many, this applies not only to the items we buy, but also to the service that we receive in the process. Some shops, such as the independent boutiques have always offered a very personal service, but now chain stores and department stores have also realised that the shopper needs and wants help and advice. This service is free, so find out if it's available in the shop of your choice. You are not obligated to buy what a shop assistant suggests (many are on commission), but often valuable advice may be given.

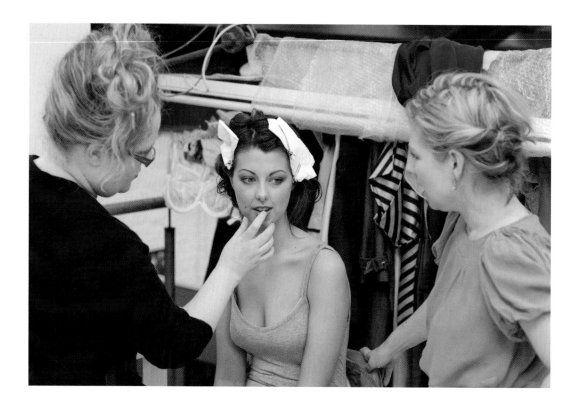

E.G. DUNNES STORES, PENNEYS, T.K. MAXX, ETC.

The value department store is a very valuable resource for anyone looking to nail a new improved style and a fully functioning wardrobe. In recent years, quality and design in these stores has improved greatly. Creating a new wardrobe is a daunting and expensive task. Your wardrobe should evolve and grow throughout your lifetime, so why not start gently with some inexpensive basics.

Things that value department stores do very well: Daywear and work-wear, such as skirts, simple tops, scarves, costume jewellery. We strongly advocate moving away from black as the cornerstone of your wardrobe. So, look for shoes in navy, grey or brown to begin expanding the possibilities of your style.

Mid-range department stores

E.G. MARKS & SPENCER, ARNOTTS, DEBENHAMS, ETC.

In fashion retailing terms, these are the true workhorses. A mid-range department store can cater for any ocassion, from a walk in the park to a walk down the aisle. What we like about these stores is that they represent true value for money. They offer strong in-house collections at affordable prices. For a slightly greater investment than you would make in the lower end department store, you can buy gar-ments which will give you enduring use. You are shopping for well-cut basic elements, the backbone of your wardrobe.

Things that the mid-range department stores do best: Trousers, jackets, coats, accessories, dresses. Occasion wear is often very well represented (Debenhams, particularly, carry an excellent range from size 6 to size 22).

High-end department stores
E.G. BROWN THOMAS, HARVEY NICHOLS, ETC.

The high-end department store is a beautiful window into the world of high fashion and luxury goods. It's safe to say that most of the departments in these great elegant stores are aimed at an elite section of society, but anyone can take inspiration from their beautiful displays. If you are already a customer, or have the budget to fill your wardrobe from these stores, by all means, go for it. Make sure, however, that you receive the service you are paying for.

What the high-end department store does best: It is a joy in itself to luxuriate in the top fashion collections of the season. Consider it a theatre of sorts. It is also great research into how the high street chains design their collections around the heavy-hitting design houses. 'Heirloom pieces', although not necessarily expensive, can be found in abundance here. If the budget is there, key items to go for are: shoes, jackets, classic dresses (not ones that are going to sit unused in the back of your wardrobe), and accessories.

The high-end department store really bears fruit at sale time, as a rarefied world is opened up to all of us. Classic buys are usually the first to be snapped up, but keep your eyes peeled for items that fit into your grand plan. It's only a bargain if you would have lusted after it at full price. More importantly, it's only a bargain if you will wear it.

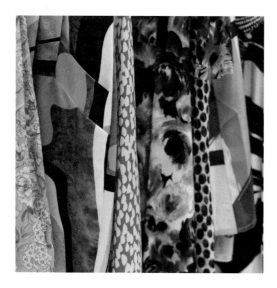

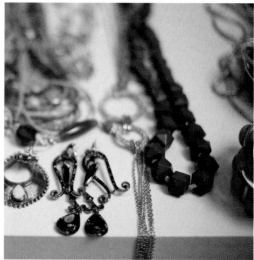

High street chains
E.G. WALLIS, OASIS, TOPSHOP, WAREHOUSE, H&M, ZARA, A·WEAR, ETC.

161

The high street chain store has become a major feature of our shopping landscape in the last ten years. Many European main streets glow with the logos of the shops above. They provide us with a very important resource. These stores are the best at picking up and interpreting up to the minute fashion trends. Topshop now shows its own collection at London Fashion Week, alongside Paul Smith, Nicole Farhi and Vivienne Westwood. What we can get from these stores is a little fashion fix without massive investment. Our wardrobes and our lives would be very boring without an occasional injection of fun. If the world's top designers decree that leopard skin print is the order of the day, our advice is to wait for the chain stores to reproduce it. Big and bold becomes tiresome quickly. But that does not mean it's not fun while it lasts.

What high street chain stores do best: Trends, colour, pattern, unusual shapes, jewellery, shoes and accessories.

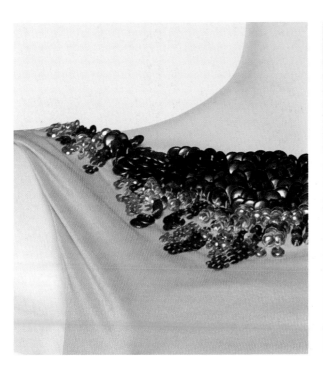
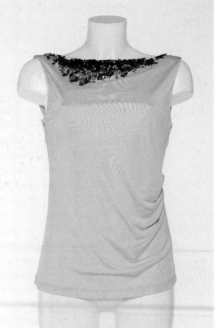

Independent boutiques

There are hundreds of interesting independent boutiques scattered throughout the country.

We have a special place in our hearts for these guys. These independent fashion stores have a big battle to fight. They are often trailblazers, seeking out and championing new designers, before the bigger guys have either heard of them or are willing to invest.

When independent boutiques are really good, they offer excellent personal service, exclusive designs and clever head to toe collections. Independent boutiques survive by building relationships with their clientele, and can often offer a full styling service. As a result, the phrase 'boutique atmosphere' has been adopted by the big guns, as they attempt to emulate what the independents nailed so long ago.

What independent boutiques do best: Smart casual outfits built by layering, occasion wear and coats.

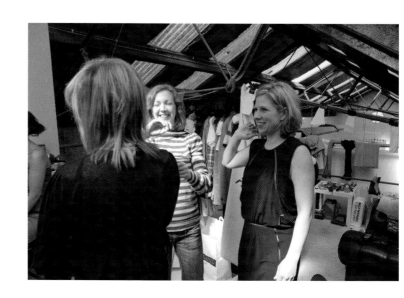

Every city has its hidden vintage purveyors.

Vintage stores are the individualist's dream. Where else can you be guaranteed a unique piece of fashion history for a small investment? Vintage can be difficult to pull off, unless you know what you're doing. Dip your toe in with accessories and don't feel tempted to go head to toe vintage. The way to make it work is by integrating selected pieces into a contemporary wardrobe. Vintage stores are also a really good source for research. If an item looks stylish after 30, 40 or 50 years, chances are it will look good in another 50 – now that's investment buying! Interestingly, if you look for classic vintage silhouettes and detailing in contemporary clothes, you can be pretty sure that they will have a healthy lifespan in your wardrobe.

One thing to be aware of when buying vintage is that an item that may have been unworn for decades can go into shock at being moved, and delicate fabrics have a habit of disintegrating before your very eyes.

Outlets

It's an appealing concept – vast expanses of 'designer' clothes at knockdown prices. The outlet is not for the fainthearted, and we would suggest waiting until you've mastered the basics before diving into these choppy waters. Many outlet stores are stocked with fillers (cheap merchandise masquerading as a bargain).

All that said, some serious gems have been unearthed, but it takes fortitude and a keen eye.

What outlets do best: Shoes, bags and jewellery are easy to buy at outlets, because they are easy to pick up and try on.

Swap shops

Often found in affluent areas, the swap shop can be a treasure trove of designer finds. Equally, if you have a wardrobe full of expensive clothes that you never wear, seek out one of these and you may get a rebate on your bad buys or put their value against something you prefer. You will always need perseverance with a swap shop, as the owner has little control over the stock they carry. Don't go expecting to find treasure, but revel in your success if you do.

Charity shops

In these straitened times, the charity shop has been reborn. Particular stores specialise in vintage or wedding collections. If you're in the mood for some charity shopping (maybe while you're donating some un-wanted items yourself), look on it as a bit of fun, and when you see something that interests you, put an extra zero onto the price – would you still buy it? If not, put it down and walk away.

Markets

Markets are a great day out. They are also a brilliant breeding ground for new talent. Many young designers start with a stall, as it is so difficult to price accessibly for retail mark-up. Also, a new brand of fashion car-boot sales see style savvy hoarders offloading their excess baggage.

The internet

The internet provides a world of infinite possibilities for success and failure.

Today's shopping landscape has been dramatically broadened by the advent and success of internet shopping. It took a while to catch on and hasn't reached its peak yet. Retail analysts predict that the market will grow by over 130 per cent over the next four years. The hunt can be daunting.

However, the internet provides a very important resource for a very simple reason.

Traditional retailers have huge overheads to outlay and every square inch must be full of merchandise with the broadest appeal so that profits can be made. This means that the 'sizing window' tends to be 8 to 18 for clothing, and 37 to 41 for footwear. Everyone knows that there are plenty of women out there both smaller and bigger than this. The problem is that they are in a minority, and so are not considered a profitable target market.

It's terrible to think that you can be made to feel invalidated simply by your clothes size, but it's all down to economics at the end of the shopping day. Step in, internet shopping – when you take away the burden of staffing and premises costs, and globalise your potential market, new possibilities arise. We don't suggest that you replace traditional clothes shopping with the cursor, but as you will see in our shopping guide, it can be a great addition for 'specialist' needs.

How you choose to stock your new wardrobe is up to you, and each of the above options have their merits. A really clever shopper will combine them all to create a truly personalised style. Find what works for you to make shopping the most pleasant and effective process possible. Enjoy the ride!

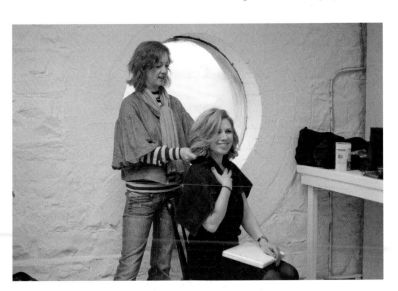

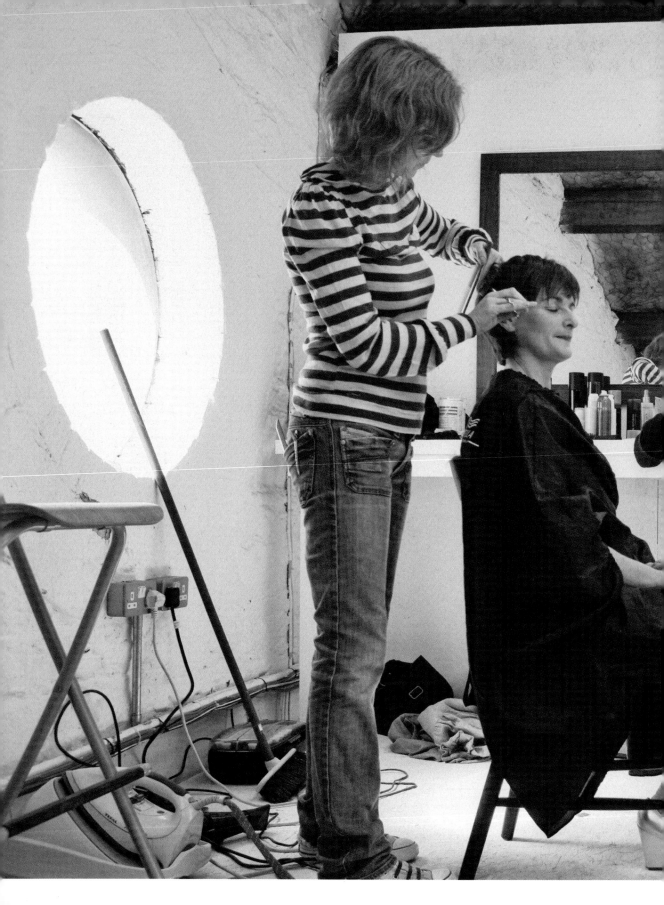

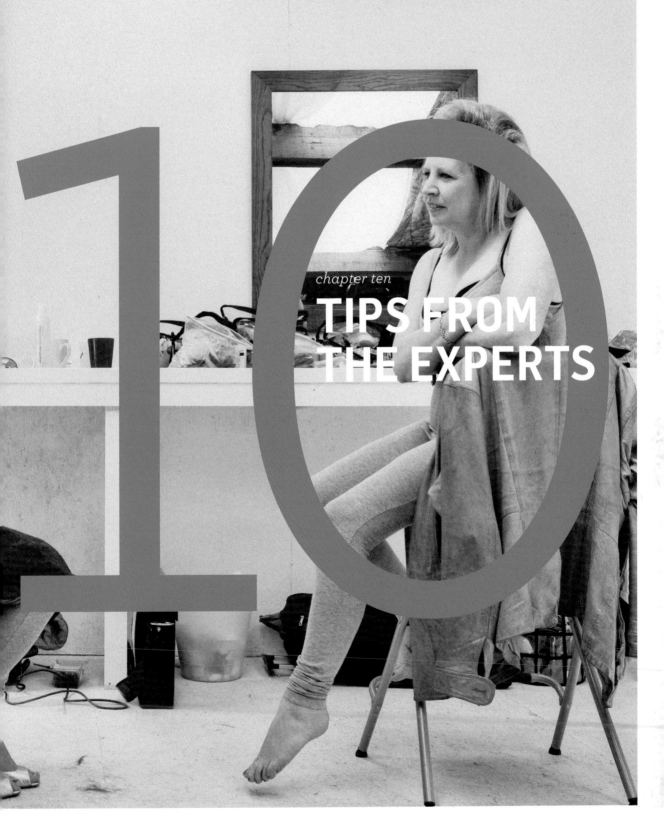

10

chapter ten

TIPS FROM THE EXPERTS

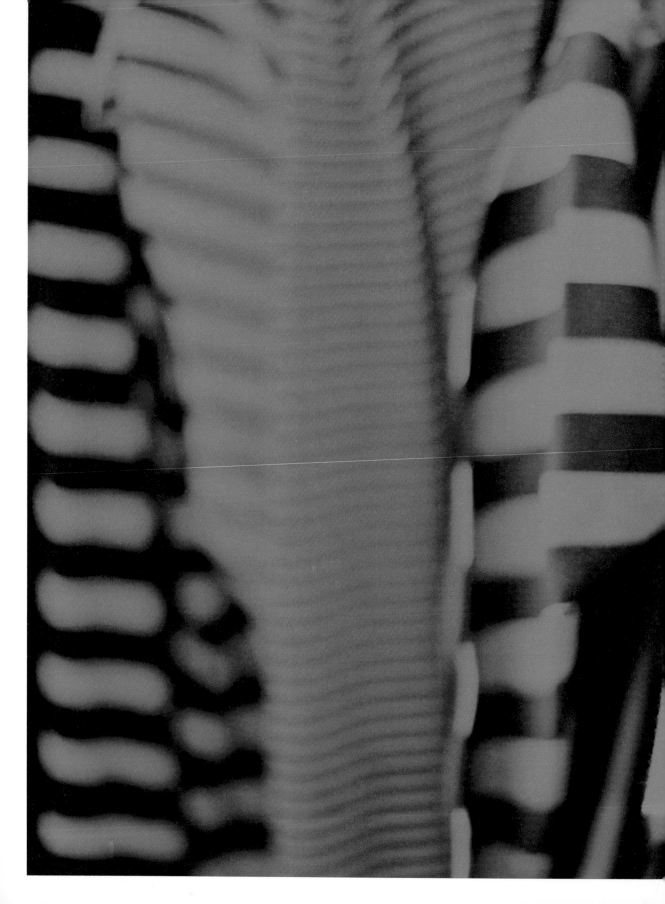

Tips from the experts

This book is our way of imparting our knowledge and experience to you, so you can discover the new you and learn to love your look. But some things are always best left to the experts – basically that means you will always need a professional to re-measure your bust accurately, to cut and style your hair, and to give you advice on skincare and how to apply your make-up.

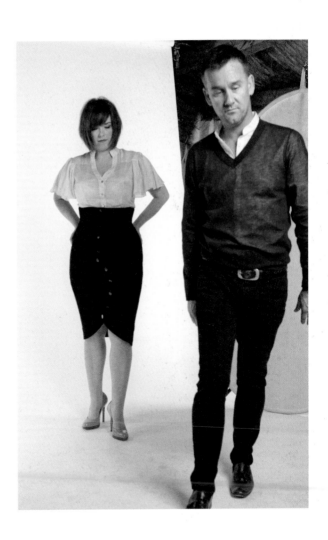

Bra measuring

Whenever we begin a transformation with one of our ladies, we always start at the same point. In order to look good in your clothes, everything must be in the right place. For this you need to be wearing the right size bra. It's impossible to see the true line of the torso when your boobs are in the way. We can't believe the number of women out there who are wearing ill-fitting bras. Once you are re-fitted the benefits are obvious; your breasts look more pert, your back looks straighter, and your tummy appears smaller. The most important thing is to find an expert that you trust. Commercially available bra sizes range from 28A to 56FF, but generally stores stock 30A to 40G. If you are larger or smaller than these sizes, the internet can be your best friend.

We are pretty good at measuring our girls, but even we seek a second opinion, because of the overall impact of the correct bra size on our transformations.

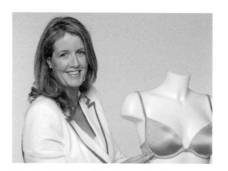

Clodagh Weber, 'knicker picker'

Clodagh Weber Knicker Picker

I work with women of all shapes and sizes and I know how difficult many of you find it to get a bra that fits perfectly, and makes you feel good too. These are the most common questions I am asked:

- How do I know if my bra is fitting me properly?
- Why are my breasts sagging?
- Why is the back of the bra rising up my back?
- Why am I spilling out of the cup?
- Why is the cup digging into my breasts?
- Why do I have this back fat?
- Why do I have big ridges on my shoulders?

All these problems are very common and are all very easily resolved. I would always say that one of the most important things to do when buying clothes would be to get professionally fitted for a bra first. A proper-fitting bra makes a huge difference to the way you look. It can take pounds off you and improve your silhouette.

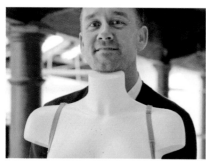

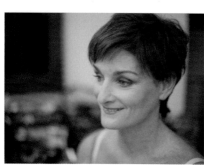

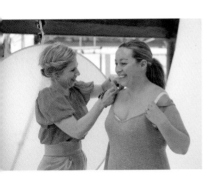

- If a bra is fitting correctly, the band will fit firmly around the back (not too tight) and the cup will fit completely around the breast (not digging in at all). So you should not have any of the problems mentioned.

- The main reason why breasts will sag is because the band of the bra is too loose. Try a band size smaller, but when you do this, go up a cup size.

- A bra that rises up your back is far too big around the band – the band is the measurement around your back, 34, 36, 38, etc. Try a back size smaller again and go up a cup size.

- When someone is spilling out of a bra, this is because the cup size is too small. The cup measurement is the size of your breast, B, C, D, etc. Try a bigger cup size, one or two letters up.

- When the cup is digging into your breast, this is also because the cup is too small. Try one or two cup sizes bigger.

- Back fat is a problem for a lot of ladies – some people think by going up a back size, this solves the problem, but it usually makes it worse. If it is really noticeable, try a bra with a wider band on the back, but make sure not to go too loose around the back, as this is the primary source of the bra's support.

- Ridges are caused when a bra either has very little support in the underwire or no wire at all. A bra's secondary support is in the underwire, not in the straps. Some people think that a really good supportive bra has to have really wide straps – this is not the case at all. The underwire is where much of the support is given, so make sure to get a really good underwire bra when you are being fitted.

(The only occasions when I would advise you not to wear an underwire bra, is when pregnant, breastfeeding or for sports use.)

All these answers are guidelines – getting professionally fitted is really the most important thing for all women, regardless of their shape or size.

Clodagh Weber at **Bramora** (www.bramora.com)

Make-up: 'the final frontier'

Many women are afraid to experiment with their make-up, but surprisingly, many more don't even know where to start. We love make-up – it can change your look in an instant. We try and break our gals out of what we call 'the look trap', which is when women get stuck in a rut and they wear the same make-up out of habit. Well girls, it's only make-up not cosmetic surgery. There are no risks, so dive in and experiement, with of course, the best professional help …

Christine Lucignano Face Painter

From celebrity faces to politicians, and every type of model, I have worked on them all. But I can honestly say that my favourite canvas is the 'real woman'. This is the everyday girl, who is looking to learn how to do her own make-up.

SKIN FIRST
The bottom line is that your make-up will only look as good as your skin does. Getting the skincare right will improve the appearance and overall effect of your make-up.

So, I believe that if the skin is perfected then the rest is a breeze. In the end what colour you do apply looks cleaner and smoother then ever before. So, make sure that in the budget you have set aside for your beauty products priority is given to your skincare, and what's left should go to the actual make-up!

A really great daily skincare regime is your goal. Add to that a 'seasonal' facial, that is, a visit to your trusted beauty therapist. This quarterly visit is to clean up your skin and prepare it for the next season. This means commiting yourself to a facial/check-up every three months. Make sure that you also have your moles and any unusual marks on the skin checked at least once a year. Because the change in a mole can be quite gradual, it is best to have your GP keep a record of this for you. Prevention is far more effective than correction.

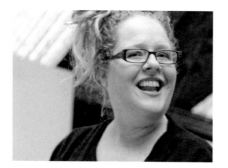
Christine Lucignano, make-up artist

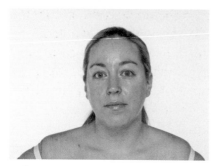
Before

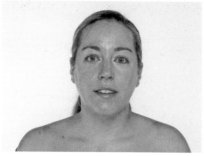
Foundation applied on the right-hand side of the face only

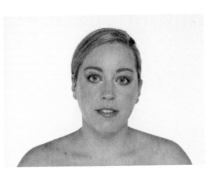

A great daytime look

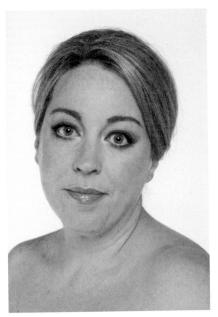

Pump up the volume for evening

FOUNDATION

The right foundation colour and finish is the basis of either good make-up or bad make-up. There are just a few rules to follow:

- Foundation is designed to do one thing – even out skin tone.
- Foundation is best used localised where there is discoloration of the skin, for instance, around the nose, mouth and chin.
- Foundation is not really intended to be used all over the entire face; simply because we are not discoloured all over our entire face.
- If you choose to apply foundation on your entire face, then the chances are that you will flatten your features and lose the fresh appearance of your skin.
- Foundation is not meant to change your skin tone!

EYE MAKE-UP

Let's face it, you're either confident with doing your eye make-up or you're not. Most of us are not. We tend to buy eyeshadows to match our outfit. This is not the best approach. I think eye make-up should be used to do two things – firstly, to enhance the shape of your eye, and secondly to get the most sparkle out of your eye colour. The method of application you choose will effect your eye shape the most. The colours you choose will do the most to bring out your actual eye colour.

THE EXTRAS

- Using the right brushes is paramount. If you take care of them you should have them a lifetime; as you would a set of fine china. It's not necessary to own too many brushes, just the right ones. Think quality not quantity.
- A good lash curler is the key to great lashes, not just the mascara!
- Buy your mascara to suit your lash type. Thickening for sparse lashes, separating for naturally clumpy lashes etc.
- Lip hydration is essential to great looking lips. If you maintain your lips then any texture of lip product will look great. Don't underestimate the power of a great red lipstick. There is the 'right' red out there for everyone!

- Self tanning should be used sparingly. Like a narcotic, it becomes an addiction. You're actually not fooling anyone at that point. Embrace your own colouring and learn how to enhance it, not erase it.

- If your budget allows it, it's a great idea to invest in a make-up lesson with a professional make-up artist to learn how to emphasise your best features, and to get the perfect look for you.

Have fun with make-up. Don't take it too seriously! And say a big thank you to Cleopatra, as she was the first to insist on having her eyeliner on at all times!

Christine Lucignano, freelance make-up artist

Expert Tips
KEN BOYLAN (BOYLAN & BALFE)

- Before applying foundation, skin needs to be smooth and clear so that the make-up will sit well on it. I would recommend exfoliation at least once a week, and a session of mircodermabrasion once or twice a year. This removes all dead skin cells.

- After that my main tip to keep skin fresh and wrinkle free is sunblock. For every day use, Clinique Superdefense SPF 25 – it's great protection, but for sunnier days La Roche Posay SPF 50+ for the face is excellent.

- After applying foundation, I feel eyebrows are the most important feature of the face. They frame the face and open the eyes. Pluck from underneath the brow, and then fill in the browline with shadow, with colour ranging from brown through to grey, depending on skin and hair colour, using a slanted brush.

- For real staying power, use a lip liner, not just around the rim of the mouth but all over, blend it in to the lip with a good oval-shape lip brush. The brush will give a good base for your lipstick. Use lipstick, as it stays on much longer then lip gloss. After you apply your lipstick, blot with plain tissue paper (like your mum used to do) then reapply, blot, and add your lip gloss. Believe me – your lipstick will stay on much longer.

- Metallic loose eye shadows look good on their own, but try putting them over black pencil, and notice how the colour comes alive. Put black pencil on your hand and pat a loose metallic powder over it. It looks electric, and is great for night time. To stop it going all over the place, take a little bit of it on the back of your hand, then with the tip of your finger pat over your eyelid, and you will find that it won't fall. Never use a brush for this, as it will go everywhere.

- Shimmer powders or liquid can look very flattering on the face for night time. They can highlight the cheek bones, even if you don't have any, and give the illusion of radiant skin. But be careful how you apply them, as too much can look sweaty. Go too close to the under eye area and they can catch in your laughter lines and highlight them, rather than your cheek bones. So when you are putting the powder on, smile, and where the wrinkles stop, you start applying the powder; just on the cheeks and maybe a little on the bridge of the nose. If you are using a liquid shimmer, pat a small amount onto the cheek. Don't rub it on, as you will remove your foundation. So, pat, pat, pat for a gorgeous shimmering glow!

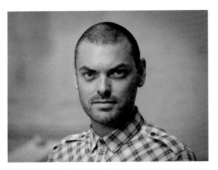

Derrick Carberry, make-up artist

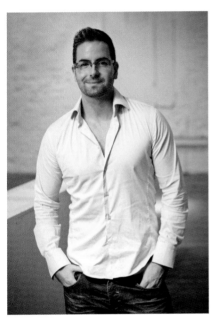

Ken Boylan, make-up artist

Expert Tips
DERRICK CARBERRY (WWW.DERRICKCARBERRY.COM)

- Brushes are the key when applying your make-up. Investing money in good quality natural-hair brushes will not only enhance the finish of products on your skin, but will minimise the amount of make-up you're using, thus saving you money in the long run. Also if you care for your brushes; carefully washing them with mild shampoo after use, your brushes can last you up to 10 years. (I still have brushes in my kit from over 12 years ago.)

- Choosing the correct foundation is so important – it conceals flaws and imperfections and evens out skin tone. Yellow/golden based foundations take down any redness in skin. Always go to a professional if you are unsure of what works for you when picking your foundation. Don't be afraid to ask as many questions as you need to, until you're satisfied that you have the correct product for you. Describe how your skin feels, for instance, dry, combination, oily or dehydrated. Ask to take away a small sample to try at home, before you commit to buying the product. Also our skin changes from season to season, so you may need to use different foundations in summer and winter.

- Eyeliner is an important element of eye make-up – it can accentuate the eye, change its shape and make the eyelashes appear thicker. Eye lining techniques can vary depending on the eye shape and desired look.

  Almond shape: line the eye from the inner corner, gradually thickening and tapering the liner towards the outer corner. To lengthen and exaggerate the eye, extend the line slightly from the outer corner.

  Round shape: line the eye from the inner corner, gradually thickening the line towards the centre of the eye to create height, and then tapering the line at the outer corner to achieve an 'open-eyed' look.

- Mascara – 'Don't leave home without it'. It creates the illusion of thicker, longer and darker eyelashes, and enhances the shape of the eye and complements its colour. Different coloured mascaras are a great way of bringing out eye colour, and are lots of fun. Stroke the lashes with the wand to apply a layer of mascara to build thickness and length, stroking away from the eye. I love using the wand tip to really separate the lashes and create a fanned effect.

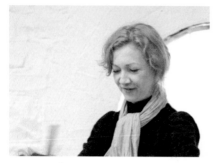

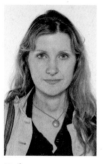

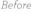

Zara Cox, hair messer

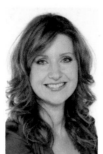

Before   *After*

Your crowning glory

Your hair should be your crowning glory. A good cut and colour can take years off you. We suggest finding a good hairdresser and sticking with them, as it is important to have a good rapport with him or her.

Zara Cox Hair Messer

THE BASICS

I believe that investing in a good cut and colour is essential. Always insist on a consultation and come prepared. I love when clients bring pictures, good and bad, they speak a thousand words, and let us know your likes and dislikes. Your hair should fit your lifestyle's needs; if you are a low maintenance girl, don't stray too far from your natural hair colour or pick a look or cut that requires a lot of work. Heed professional advice, especially when it comes to suitability. I, and other good hair stylists, will happily talk about your hair all day, so next time you're getting your hair done, come early and take advantage of that. Always ask for tips on products and alternative ways to dress your hair.

PRODUCTS

I feel it is really important to seek professional advice when buying products – who doesn't have loads of unused magic potions cluttering up their bathrooms? Product technology is the fastest moving aspect of hairdressing, and with so much time and money going into research, the right products can really improve the look and feel of your hair. The list is endless when it comes to what a product can do for your hair – modern products tackle everything from UV protection to humidity, as well as providing quick rinse formulas, wearable treatments and a variety of hold factors. There is even a new hair straightening system which gives healthy shiny hair.

Looking at a shelf packed with every type of hair product can be bewildering, so it's best to seek advice from a professional, who will analyse your hair and its needs, and point you in the right direction to maintain, moisturise and strengthen your hair.

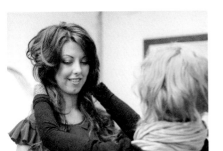

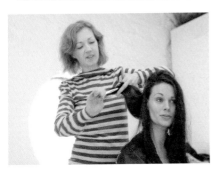

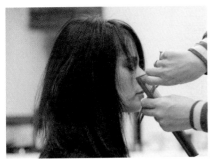

Modern products can put you in total control of your hair. You'll need different products for your hair, depending on whether you're styling it for every day, or going out. Every day maintenance depends on how much time you have – choose a product to suit your hair type to get the best result. If you're styling your hair for a night out, have fun with it! This is where hair products can really work their magic, and you can change the natural texture of your hair, whether you want to go wild or go for a classic style.

Hair tools

Invest in the best quality tools that you can afford. Your essential kit should contain:

- A hairdryer: Should be lightweight, have a variety of heat and speed settings and a nozzle.
- Ceramic straighteners: Make sure it has heat-controlled settings and rounded edges.
- Heated rollers: Should be ceramic and in a variety of sizes. Using a set with claws rather than pins, as they make the job easier.
- Tongs: Heat controlled settings are essential. Use whatever size barrel suits your needs.
- Brushes: Natural bristles with a ceramic barrel are best. Although the type of brushes you need depend on your hairstyle, the Marilyn Teaser backcombing brush is a must in my kit.
- Straight hairpins, Kirby grips, and hair bungees.

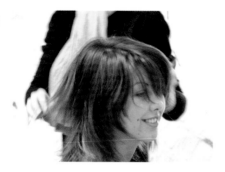

Putting your hair up

Preparation is key to putting your hair up quickly and easily. Start off with shampooing that morning, and blast dry using a texturising product like mousse. Even if you are wearing your hair smooth, light backcombing is the foundation to all up-styles. Don't open your hairclips to use them, as it forces too much hair into the clip, and pushes it back out. When putting hair up, try to keep your head in a natural upright position. To build up texture, rather than wetting your hair, use short blasts of hairspray, not too close to the head. Practise putting up your hair before your night out. Be brave – even small changes can have a massive impact. Changing your parting or adding some curl or texture can transform your look. Above all, have fun – go for it!

Zara Cox at **Queen Beauty Emporium** (www.queenbe.ie)

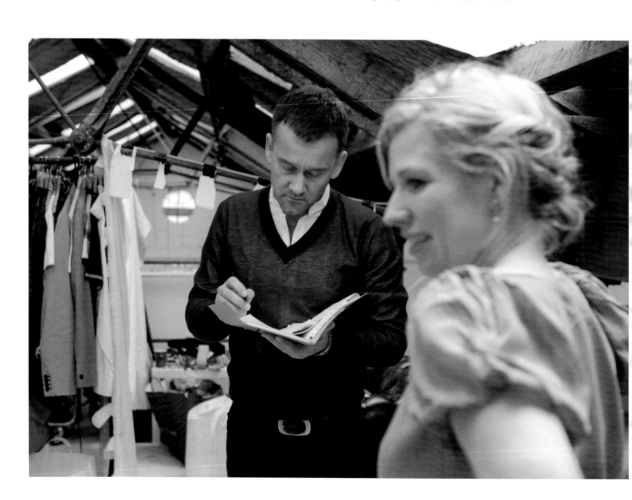

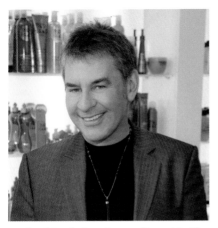

Michael Doyle, hairdresser (Peter Mark)

Expert Tips

MICHAEL DOYLE, INTERNATIONAL SESSION HAIRDRESSER FOR PETER MARK

- What is hair? Hair is made up of a dead protein called keratin. However, the follicles nestling just below your scalp are very much alive and need nourishment. The best nourishment hair can get comes from food; a diet rich in protein, zinc, copper and vitamin A is perfect for healthy locks. So tuck into a big juicy steak and plenty of dark green vegetables!

- Hair stress test: We are constantly putting our hair under stress. Dieting, chemical treatments, and day to day living can become a relentless onslaught on our locks. To test whether your hair is healthy or not, try this simple test; drop a strand of your hair into water and give it a little tap with your finger. If it floats, congratulations, your hair is healthy! If it sinks, your hair is dry or damaged.

- Treatments: There are two very different types of treatment available to improve the health of your hair. Conditioning treatments will add moisture and sleekness, and protein ones will add volume. When using either, leave on for at least two minutes, so that your hair can absorb the nutrients. Rinse for twice as long as usual to get rid of any residue, and resist the temptation to towel dry your hair too vigorously.

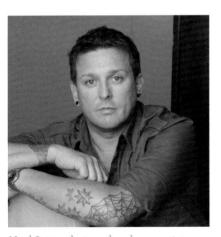

Noel Sutton, hair and make-up artist

Expert Tips

NOEL SUTTON, FREELANCE HAIR AND MAKE-UP ARTIST

- Styling: The wonderful thing about hair is that, with even a small change, you can add a new lease of life to your style. Try changing your parting, cutting a fringe or altering the shade, or be brave and go for a new style altogether.

- Have fun with your hair. Experiment at home; dig out your heated rollers, dust off the curling tongs and plug in your straightening irons. Whether you go for soft waves, slinky straight or an elegant upstyle, you can create a new look at home without spending a penny.

- Washing: Make sure to brush out any tangles before you wash your hair. It is better to use warm rather than hot water. If the temperature is too hot, it may dry out your scalp and cause itchiness. If you have oily hair, hot water will make the oil glands overreact and exacerbate the problem. Always make sure to rinse your hair well, and use cool water for the final rinse. This will help to give shine to your lovely locks.

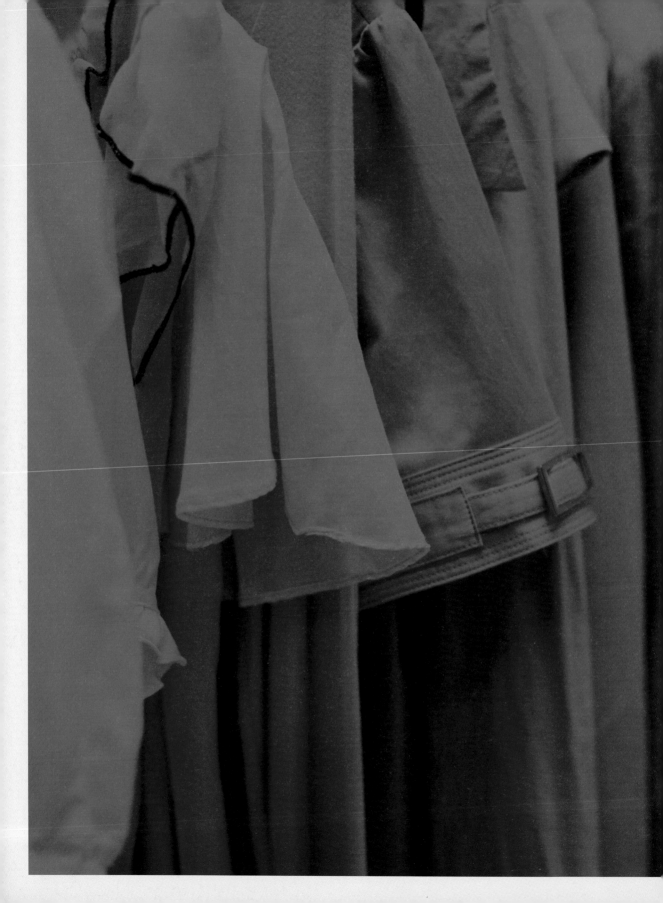

SHOPPING GUIDE

To make your shopping easier, we've included this guide to get you started. Happy shopping!

Value department stores

Dunnes Stores
Nationwide
www.dunnestores.ie

Pennys
Nationwide
www.primark.co.uk

T.K. Maxx
Nationwide
www.tkmaxx.com

Mid-range department stores

Arnotts
Henry Street, Dublin 1.
T 01 8050400
www.buy4now.ie/arnottsstore

Clerys
18–27 Lower O'Connell Street, Dublin 1.
T 01 8786000
www.clerys.ie

Debenhams
Nationwide
www.debenhams.com

Marks & Spencer
Nationwide
www.marks&spencer.com

High-end department stores

Brown Thomas
· Grafton Street, Dublin 2.
  T 01 6056666
· Patrick Street, Cork.
  T 021 4805555

· O'Connell Street, Limerick.
  T 061 417222
· Eglington Street, Galway.
  T 091 565254
www.brownthomas.com

Harvey Nichols
Dundrum Town Centre, Dublin 16.
T 01 2910488
www.harveynichols.com

House of Fraser
Dundrum Town Centre, Dublin 16.
T 01 2991400
www.houseoffraser.co.uk

Chain stores

A|Wear
Nationwide
www.awear.com

Barratts
Nationwide
www.barratts.co.uk

BT2
· 180–181 The Red Mall,
  Blanchardstown Centre,
  Dublin 15. T 01 8606540
· Unit 133, Dundrum Town Centre,
  Dublin 16. T 01 2968400
· 28–29 Grafton Street, Dublin 2.
  T 01 6056747
www.bt2.ie

Coast
Nationwide
www.coast-stores.com

Dorothy Perkins
Nationwide
www.dorothyperkins.com

Evans (Great for bigger girls!)
Nationwide
www.evans.co.uk

Fitzpatrick Shoes
· 76 Grafton Street, Dublin 2.
  T 01 6772333
· Unit 3, Dundrum Town Centre,
  Dublin 16. T 01 2983270
· Units 5/6 Custom House Quay,
  IFSC, Dublin 1. T 01 8590370
www.fitzpatricksshoes.com

Fran & Jane
· 2a Main Street, Blackrock, Co. Dublin.
  T 01 2108539
· 22 Oliver Plunkett, Co. Cork.
  T 021 4279598
· 1 Market House, Market Street,
  Clonmel, Co. Tipperary. T 052 70040
· Unit 2, Lesley Plaza, Lisburn Road,
  Belfast. T 028 90687716
www.franandjane.ie

French Connection
Nationwide
www.frenchconnection.com

Genius Denim Specialists
· 6a Powerscourt Townhouse Centre,
  Dublin 2. T 01 6797851
· The Gallery, Dundrum Town Centre,
  Dublin 16. T 01 2962992
· Swan Centre, Rathmines, Dublin 6.
  T 01 4961566
www.genius.ie

H&M
Nationwide
www.h&m.com/ie

Karen Millen
Nationwide
www.karenmillen.com

Miss Selfridge
- 18/27 Lower O'Connell Street, Dublin 1. T 01 8786000
- Liffey Valley Shopping Centre, Dublin 22. T 01 6234666
- Patrick Street, Cork. T 021 4277727
- Unit 224, Blanchardstown Centre, Dublin 15. T 01 8222192
- Unit 2/3, Galway Shopping Centre, Galway. T 091 567367
- Unit 468, Jervis Shopping Centre, Dublin 1. T 01 8735390
- Unit 13/14, Letterkenny Retail Park, New Link Road, Co. Donegal. T 074 9161613

Monsoon
Nationwide
www.monsoon.co.uk

New Look
- 101 Liffey Valley Shopping Centre, Dublin 22. T 01 6235462
- Also nationwide
www.newlook.co.uk

Next
Nationwide
www.nextdirectory.ie

Oasis
Nationwide
www.oasis-stores.com

Office
- 6 Henry Street, Dublin 1. T 01 8748250
- Grafton Street, Dublin 2. T 01 6709960
- Unit 27, Liffey Valley Shopping Centre, Dublin 22. T 01 6203975
- Unit 20, Dundrum Town Centre, Dublin 16. T 01 2963381
www.office.co.uk

Pamela Scott
- 84 Grafton Street, Dublin 2. T 01 6796655
- Blanchardstown Centre, Dublin 15. T 01 8221507
- Frascati Centre, Blackrock, Co. Dublin. T 01 2834164
- The Pavillons Shopping Centre, Swords, Co. Dublin. T 01 8903033
- Dundrum Town Centre, Dublin 16. T 01 2983246
- 9 Fairgreen Centre, Co. Carlow. T 059 9182304

- Scotch Hall, Drogheda, Co. Louth. T 041 9802462
- Bridgewater, Arklow, Co. Wicklow. T 0402 41042
- Oliver Plunkett Street, Cork. T 021 4273759
- The Crescent Centre, Dooradoyle, Limerick. T 061 774380
- John Roberts Square, Strand Street, Waterford. T 051 874844
- Central Plaza, Abbeycourt, Tralee, Co. Kerry. T 066 7193053
- Mahon Point Shopping Centre, Cork. T 021 4536620
www.pamelascott.ie

Reiss
1 Stephen's Green Street, Dublin 2. T 01 6712588
www.reiss.co.uk

River Island
Nationwide
www.riverisland.com

Schuh
Nationwide
www.schuh.co.uk

Topshop
Nationwide
www.topshop.com

United Colours of Benetton
Nationwide
www.benetton.com

Wallis
Nationwide
www.wallis-fashion.com

Warehouse
Nationwide
www.warehouse.ie

Zara
Nationwide
www.zara.com

Vintage and antique clothing

A Store is Born
34 Clarendon Street, Dublin 2. T 01 6795866

The Accidental Boutique
(By appointment only)
102 Kincora Road, Clontarf, Dublin 3. M 087 2319656
www.accidentalboutique.com

Dirty Fabulous
97 Lower Baggot Street, Dublin 2. T 01 6624249

Enchanted Vintage Clothing
Benbulben Centre, Rathcormac, Co. Sligo. T 071 9146680
www.vintageclothing.ie

The Goddess Room
Unit 5 Theatre Lane, Greystones, Co. Wicklow. T 087 2739203
www.thegoddessroom.net

Harlequin
13 Castle Market, Dublin 2. T 01 6710202

Jenny Vander
Drury Street, Dublin 2. T 01 6770406

Lucy's Lounge
11 Foynes Street, Temple Bar, Dublin 2.
www.lucyslounge-deeblogspot.com

Wild Child
61 South Great Georges Street, Dublin 2. T 01 4755099

Independent boutiques
Connaught

Belle Blu
Market Street, Clifden, Co. Galway. T 095 21321
www.belleblu.com

Cinders Shoe Heaven
16 Upper Abbeygate Street, Co. Galway. T 091 533696
www.cinders.ie

Cobblers Shoes
Dunkellian Street, Loughrea, Co. Galway. T 091 870244

Cobwebs
7 Quay Lane, Galway. T 091 564 38853
www.cobwebs.ie

Collette Latchford
Lyndon Court, Galway. T 091 563630

Demora
Cross Street, Galway. T 091 539860

Design Platform
The Courtyard, Clifden Station House, Co. Galway. T 091 21526

Designhouse Barna
Barna Village Centre, Co. Galway. T 091 596000

The Green Room
10 Pearse Road, Co. Sligo. T 071 9150950

Kaizen Boutique
Bridge Street, Carrick-on-Shannon,
Co. Leitrim. T 071 9650746

La Femme
29 O'Connell Street, Co. Sligo.
T 071 9143331

Les Jumelles
11 Upper Abbeygate Street, Galway
T 091 564540

Liberties
The Quay, Westport, Co. Mayo.
T 098 50273
www.liberties.ie

Marann
Teeling Street, Tubbercurry, Co. Sligo.
T 071 9120898

McGuire Shoes
• Ellison Street, Castlebar, Co. Mayo.
  T 094 9028999
• Tone Street, Ballina, Co. Mayo.
  T 096 21363
www.mcguireshoes.com

Meg
Mount Street, Claremorris, Co. Mayo.
T 094 9377738
www.megshops.com

Monet
Dunkellin Street, Loughrea, Co. Galway.
T 091 841911

Myriam O'Reilly
7 Eyre Street, Galway. T 091 561866

Okinara House of Fashion
Moycullen, Co. Galway. T 091 555755

Pagan
48 Upper Abbeygate Street, Galway.
T 091 569767

Passenger
Clifden Station House Courtyard,
Clifden, Co. Galway. T 095 22770

Premoli
William Street, Galway. T 091 566087

Regis
9 Lower Abbeygate Street, Galway.
T 091 569696

Rococo
Cross Street, Galway. T 091 565856

Select
2–3 Lismoyle House, Augustine Street,
Galway. T 091 532629

Stephanie Lynch Boutique
39 Eyre Street, Galway. T 091 566383

Style Plus
(Great occasion wear for bigger girls!)
Galway, 5 Carlycon House, Main Street,
Oranmore, Co. Galway. T 091 788750

Zodi
8 Wine Street, Sligo. T 071 9145555

Zulu
Wine Street, Sligo. T 071 9144738

Independent boutiques
Dublin

Airwaves
• Stillorgan Shopping Centre,
  Co. Dublin. T 01 2880518
• Bloomfield Shopping Centre,
  Dún Laoghaire, Co. Dublin.
  T 01 2801922
• 15 Westbury Mall, Dublin 2.
  T 01 6776321

Alila
41 Dury Street, Dublin 2. T 01 6799547
www.alila.ie

Allicano
4 Johnson's Place, Dublin 2.
T 01 6773430

Anastasia
114 Main Street, Ranelagh, Dublin 6.
T 01 4912031
www.anastasia.ie

Anthologie
51 Clontarf Road, Dublin 3. T 01 8532100

Ashley Reeves
• Stillorgan Shopping Centre,
  Co. Dublin. T 01 2886276
• Rathfarnham Shopping Centre,
  Dublin 14. T 01 4934609

Audrey Taylor
52 Sandycove Road, Co. Dublin.
T 01 2841988

Aura
94 Sandymount Road, Dublin 4.
T 01 6672377
www.aurashop.ie

Ted Baker
42 Grafton Street, Dublin 2. T 01 8814111

Barnardo Furriers
108 Grafton Street, Dublin 2.
T 01 6777867

Bella Mamma
The Triangle, Ranelagh, Dublin 6.
T 01 4968598
www.bellamamma.ie

Bibas Boutique
Main Street, Malahide, Co. Dublin.
T 01 8451529

Blue
51 Main Street, Blackrock, Co. Dublin.
T 01 2109939

Bolero
2 Railway Road, Dalkey, Co. Dublin.
T 01 2850104
www.irishboutiques.com

Bow
Unit 4, Powerscourt Centre, Dublin 2.
T 01 6040044

Buffalo
16 Exchequer, Street Dublin 2.
T 01 6712492
www.buffaloshop.de

Caru
30 Drury Street, Dublin 2. T 01 6040757
www.caru.ie

Chantelle
The Crescent, Monkstown, Co. Dublin.
T 01 2803163

Cherche Midi
23 Drury Street, Dublin 2. T 01 6753974

Chica
Westbury Mall, Dublin 2.
T 01 6719836
www.chicaboutiqueonline.com

China Pink
38 Dunville Avenue, Ranelagh, Dublin 6.
T 01 4888000
www.chinapink.ie

Cinders Shoe Heaven
• 22 Wicklow Street, Dublin 2.
  T 01 6777491
• Merrion Shopping Centre, Dublin 4.
  T 01 2837662
www.cinders.ie

Circus
Powerscourt Centre, Dublin 2.
T 01 6724736
www.circusstore.net

Claudio Ferrici
31 Westbury Mall, Dublin 2. T 01 6746662

Clothes Peg
Sutton Cross, Dublin 13. T 01 8321130

Cocobelle
Unit 25, Royal Hibernian Way,
Dublin 2. T 01 7071818
www.cocobelle.ie

Compagnie L
Merrion Centre, Dublin 4. T 01 2601580

Costume
10–11 Castle Market, Dublin 2.
T 01 6794188

Coze Di Roze
Johnstown Road, Cabinteely Village,
Dublin 18. T 01 2351305
www.cozediroze.ie

Cyan
Swan Centre, Rathmines, Dublin 6.
T 01 4968681

Design Centre
Powerscourt Centre, Dublin 2.
T 01 6795718
www.designcentre.ie

Diffusion
47 Clontarf Road, Dublin 3. T 01 8331592
www.diffusion.ie

Divine
2 Strand Street, Malahide, Co. Dublin.
T 01 8451592
www.divine.ie

Dolls
32B Clarendon Street, Dublin 2.
T 01 6729004
www.dolls.ie

Dress Circle
136 Terenure Road, Dublin 6.
T 01 4904115

Emma
33 Claredon Street, Dublin 2.
T 01 6339781
www.emma.ie

Emme
• 36 Dunville Avenue, Ranelagh,
  Dublin 6. T 01 4971771
• Dundrum Town Centre, Dublin 16.
  T 01 2989179
• 1a Westbury Mall, Clarendon Street,
  Dublin 2. T 01 6729176

• Unit 1-2 Summerhill Road, Dunboyne,
  Co. Meath. T 01 8026724
• Unit 6 Laurence Town Centre,
  Drogheda, Co. Louth. T 041 9843757
• Unit 24/25, The CHQ Building, IFSC,
  Docklands, Dublin 1. T 01 6702640

Frizzante
99a Rathgar Road, Rathgar, Dublin 6.
T 01 4903768

Halo
4a Glasthule Road, Sandycove,
Co. Dublin. T 01 2845922

Havana
2 Anglesea House, Donnybrook,
Dublin 4. T 01 2602707

Indigo and Cloth
Basement, 27 South William Street,
Dublin 2. T 01 6706403
www.indigoandcloth.com

Julien
Unit 112, Stephen's Green Shopping
Centre, Dublin 2. T 01 4751144

Just in Boutique
Tower Shopping Centre, Clondalkin
Village, Dublin 22. T 01 4570990

Kelli
45 Ranelagh Village, Ranelagh, Dublin 6.
T 01 4970077

Khan
15 Rock Hill, Main Street, Blackrock,
Co. Dublin. T 01 2781646

Kohl
Unit 20, The CHQ Building, IFSC,
Dublin 1. T 01 6360136
www.kohl.ie

Lara
• 1 Dame Lane, Dublin 2. T 01 6707951
• 15 Terenure Place, Dublin 6W.
  T 01 4991622
www.laras.ie

Lisa Perkins
Unit 44, Blackrock Centre, Co. Dublin.
T 01 2884812

Little Black Dress
Top Floor, Powerscourt Centre, Dublin 2.
T 01 7079975
www.littleblackdress.ie

Loulerie
14b Chatham Street, Dublin 2.
T 01 6724024
www.loulerie.ie

Mad Hatter
20 Lower Stephen Street, Dublin 2.
T 01 4054936
www.madhatter.com

Madison
4 Brighton Road, Foxrock, Dublin 18.
T 01 2894209

Maria Fusco
38 Clarendon Street, Dublin 2.
T 01 6334712

Marian Gale
8 The Mall, Donnybrook, Dublin 4.
T 01 2697460
www.mariangale.ie

Misamu
Brighton Road, Foxrock, Dublin 18.
T 01 2897938

Miss E
57 Glasthule Road, Sandycove,
Co. Dublin. T 01 280 9849

Monica John
1 South Anne Street, Dublin 2.
T 01 6790045
www.monicajohn.com

Nelo Maternity
39 Claredon Street, Dublin 2.
T 01 6791336
www.nelomaternity.com

Neola@Malahide
Main Street, Malahide, Co. Dublin.
T 01 8456033
www.neola.ie

Noa Noa
Unit 18, Westbury Mall, Dublin 2.
T 01 7071812

Pace
3 Brighton Road, Foxrock, Dublin 18.
T 01 2897658
www.paceoffoxrock.ie

Paolo Rossi Design
• 49 Clontarf Road, Dublin 3.
  T 01 8330003
• 5 Townyard Lane, Malahide,
  Co. Dublin. T 01 8455952

Potrero Hill
Royal Hibernian Way, Dublin 2.
T 01 6330133
www.potrerohill-shop.com

Rebecca Davis
Unit 27, Westbury Mall, Dublin 2.
T 01 7645694

Richard Alan
84 Grafton Street, Dublin 2.
T 01 6165694

Rocco
196 Clontarf Road, Dublin 3.
T 01 8530299

Rococo
• Westbury Mall, Dublin 2. T 01 6704007
• 29 Glasthule Road, Sandycove,
  Co. Dublin. T 01 2300686

Sabotage
Exchequer St, Dublin 2.
T 01 6778713

Sandz
• 23 Dunville Avenue, Ranelagh,
  Dublin 6. T 01 4126514
• 34 Main Street, Blackrock, Co. Dublin.
  T 01 2108545

Sans Souci
The Green, Malahide, Co. Dublin.
T 01 8457630

Seagreen
11a–12a Monkstown Crescent,
Co. Dublin. T 01 2020130
www.seagreen.ie

Select Boutique
3 Farmhill Road, Goatstown, Dublin 14.
T 01 2982073

Serena Boutique
• Unit 3 Sandymount Road, Dublin 4.
  T 01 6676108
• Frascati Centre, Blackrock, Co. Dublin.
  T 01 2781050

Smock
31 Drury Street, Dublin 2.
T 01 6139000

Soul Designs
• 2 Glasthule Road, Sandycove,
  Co. Dublin. T 01 2808895

Stepz Shoe Boutique
Main Street, Malahide, Co. Dublin.
T 01 8456883
www.stepz.ie

Susan Hunter Lingerie
13 Westbury Mall, Dublin 2.
T 01 6791271
www.susanhunter.ie

The Turret
2–3 Castlemarket, Dublin 2.
T 01 6714936

The Wardrobe
Unit 6, Killiney Shopping Centre,
Killiney, Co. Dublin. T 01 2859616

Thomas Patrick Shoes
77 Grafton Street, Dublin 2.
T 01 6713866

Tiger Lily
Unit 4 Tyrellstown Town Centre,
Dublin 15. T 01 8272401
www.tlily.com

Transpire
Unit 7, Sutton Cross Shopping Centre,
Dublin 13. T 01 8322234
www.transpire.ie

Tres Chic
2a Main Street, Malahide, Co. Dublin.
T 01 8450139

Tulle
28 Market Arcade, South Great
George's Street, Dublin 2. T 01 6799115
www.tulledublin.com

Tyrrell & Brennan
13 Lower Pembroke Street, Dublin 2.
T 01 6788332
www.tyrrellbrennan.com

Venezuela
86 Strand Street, Skerries, Co. Dublin.
T 01 8490982

Independent boutiques
Leinster

A Touch of Class
10–11 Pearse Street, Athlone,
Co. Westmeath. T 090 6498355
www.atouchofclass.ie

An Siopa Brog
9 Castle Street, Enniscorthy,
Co. Wexford. T 053 9234546

Aria Boutique
7 Poplar Square, Naas, Co. Kildare.
T 045 871333
www.ariaboutique.ie

Ashanti Gold
• Esmonde Street, Gorey, Co. Wexford.
  T 053 9420342
• Meridian Point, Greystones,
  Co. Wicklow. T 01 2871789

Baronessa
Leinster Street, Athy, Co. Kildare.
T 059 8638720

Bella
67 Narrow West Street, Drogheda,
Co. Louth. T 041 9834047

Berry Boutique
49 Kieran Street, Co. Kilkenny.
T 056 7762177

Bijou Lingerie
14 Dublin Street, Co. Longford.
T 043 42944
www.bijou.ie

Blonde Gemini
23 The Quay, New Ross, Co. Wexford.
T 051 448750

Brass Rail
86-87 Clanbrassil Street, Dundalk,
Co. Louth. T 042 9330303

Burgess of Athlone
1–7 Church Street, Athone,
Co. Westmeath. T 090 6472005
www.burgessofathlone.ie

Butik
14a Cutlery Road, Newbridge,
Co. Kildare. T 045 435256

Caza Choo Shoe Boutique
72 High Street, Co. Kilkenny.
T 056 7790592

Chantelle
The Gables, Dunshaughlin, Co. Meath.
T 01 8259943

Choo Couture
5 Custume Place, Athlone,
Co. Westmeath. T 090 6474357

Cinders Shoe Heaven
Courtyard Shopping Centre,
Newbridge, Co. Kildare. T 045 437750

Clara Ellen
• 49 Dublin Street, Longford. T 043 48361
• 33 Church Street, Athlone,
  Co. Westmeath. T 090 6474992
• 1 Castle Street, Mullingar,
  Co. Westmeath. T 044 934 4255

Classic FX
• Meridian Point Shopping Centre,
  Greystones, Co. Wicklow.
  T 01 2871801
• Esmonde Street, Gorey, Co. Wexford.
  T 053 9420476

CoCo Pink
7 William Street, Co. Kilkenny.
T 056 7703705

Contra Clothing
99 Main Street, Gorey, Co. Wexford.
T 053 9420189

Crave Boutique
1 Castle Buildings, Friary Road, Naas,
Co. Kildare. T 045 883424

Design Platform
Marriott Johnstown House & Spa,
Enfield, Co. Meath. T 046 9540081

Divine
Unit 3 Manor Mills Shopping Centre,
Maynooth, Co. Kildare. T 01 6292550
www.divine.ie

Edel's Boutique
Unit 2 Kelton House, Lyster Square,
Portlaoise, Co. Laois. T 057 8660059
www.edelsboutique.com

Eden
No 3 Market Square, Dundalk,
Co. Louth. T 042 9386739
www.edenireland.com

Elaine Curtis
122 Tullow Street, Co. Carlow.
T 059 9141790
www.elainecurtis.ie

Emporium Kalu
16 South Main Street, Naas,
Co. Kildare. T 045 896222

Erre Esse
• Mount Wolseley Hotel, Tullow,
  Co. Carlow. T 059 9180117
• Main Street, Portlaoise, Co. Laois.
  T 057 8682375

Escape
Church Road, Greystones,
Co. Wicklow. T 01 2871524

Fabiani
12 Grafton Court, Longford.
T 043 46049

Fabucci
10 The Moat Mall, Naas, Co. Kildare.
T 045 874721

Fishers
The Old Schoolhouse,
Newtownmountkennedy, Co. Wicklow.
T 01 2819404
www.fishers.ie

Footloose on the Square
Fitzwilliam Square, Co. Wicklow.
T 0404 64244

French Connection
Strand Road, Rosslare, Co. Wexford.
T 053 9132189

Genevieve Cox
2 Dublin Street, Longford.
T 043 40777

Giorgio's Shoe Boutique
1 Hillside Road, Greystones,
Co. Wicklow. T 01 2017252

Glamour
26 Main Street, Enniscorthy,
Co. Wexford. T 053 9238144

Heaven Boutique
Marshes Shopping Centre, Dundalk,
Co. Louth. T 042 9351336

Heavenly
Main Street, Clane, Co. Kildare.
T 045 861719

Heels
Bridge Street, Co. Wicklow.
T 040 462516
www.heels.ie

Inspire Shoe Boutique
2 Cathedral Street, Enniscorthy,
Co. Wexford. T 053 9234804

Jenny Turner
The Village Centre, Enniskerry,
Co. Wicklow. T 01 2861899

Jenny's Boutique
• Main Street, Ashbourne, Co. Meath.
  T 01 8350782
• Main Street, Dunshaughlin, Co. Meath.
  T 01 8240058

Jo Duggan
3 William Street, Kilkenny.
T 056 7722217

Jolie Boutique
8 Key West, Custom House Quay,
Co. Wexford. T 053 9174961

Julu
La Touche Place, Greystones,
Co. Wicklow. T 01 2016723

Kabana Boutique
Unit 7 Abbeylands Centre, Clane,
Co. Kildare. T 045 892398

Kabelo Boutique
Emmet Square, Birr, Co. Offaly.
T 057 9123812

Kadee
9 Pearse Street, Athone, Co. Westmeath.
T 090 6498355

Kasura
12 Killegland Street, Ashbourne,
Co. Meath. T 01 8357913

Khan
27 Dominic Street, Mullingar,
Co. Westmeath. T 044 9396908

Kohl
4 Newgrange Mall, Slane, Co. Meath.
T 041 9809400

Lace
6 Market Court Town Hall Centre,
Main Street, Bray, Co. Wicklow.
T 01 2828560

Laura Gray Boutique
Shopping Centre, Church Road,
Tullamore, Co. Offaly. T 057 9341886

Little Miracle Maternity
1/2 La Touche Place, Greystones,
Co. Wicklow. T 01 2010102

Lure
51 Dublin Street, Co. Longford.
T 043 48484

Lynch's Ladies Boutique
Main Street, Banagher, Co. Offaly.
T 057 9151380
www.lynchfashions.com

Makaba
57 The Avenue, Whitewater Shopping
Centre, Newbridge, Co. Kildare.
T 045 432919
www.makaba.ie

Milan & Co
11 Florence Road, Bray, Co. Wicklow.
T 01 2865733
www.milan-co.com

Mimi Boutique
74 High Street, Kilkenny. T 056 7722100

Miro Shoes
2 Adelphi Mall, The Longwalk,
Dundalk, Co. Louth. T 042 9333620
www.miroshoes.net

Neola
River Lane, Dundalk, Co. Louth.
T 042 9335828
www.neola.ie

Nicola Ross
1a North Main Street, Naas, Co. Kildare.
T 045 875181

O'Briens
81 North Main Street, Wexford.
T 053 9123106

Olivia Danielle
19 Church Street, Athlone,
Co. Westmeath. T 090 6472707

Oona Conroy
120 Tullow Street, Co. Carlow.
T 059 9139777

Ottiva
2 Weafer Street, Enniscorthy,
Co. Wexford. T 053 9238840

Paula Boutique
Main Street, Leixlip, Co. Kildare.
T 01 6242711
www.paulaboutique.ie

Pamela Shoes
2 Irish Street, Ardee, Co. Louth.
T 041 6858511
www.pasmashoes.com

Pretty Woman
7 Main Street, Enniscorthy, Co. Wexford.
T 053 9230576

Ross Morgan
Yew Tree Square, Prosperous Road,
Co. Kildare. T 045 902162
www.rossmorgan.ie

Rubana
Unit 2 Hillside Road, Greystones,
Co. Wicklow. T 01 2016015
www.rubanaireland.ie

Scruples
Caspo Centre, Naas, Co. Kildare.
T 045 901734

Serena Boutique
Superquinn Shopping Centre, Carlow
Town, Co. Carlow. T 059 9143360

Serendipity Boutique
34 Kieran Street, Kilkenny.
T 056 7756839

Shabby Chic
Unit 6, Corballis Shopping Centre,
Ratoath, Co. Meath. T 01 6896297
www.shabbychic.ie

Shadore
Theatre Lane, Greystones, Co. Wicklow.
T 01 2875999

Sofina
The Village, Enniskerry, Co. Wicklow.
T 01 2046921
www.sofina.ie

Style Plus
(Great occasion wear for bigger girls!)
4 Riverview House, Dublin Road,
Celbridge, Co. Kildare. T 01 6276475

Suzan Belle
41 Kieran Street, Kilkenny.
T 056 7762889
www.suzanbelle.ie

Ten
The Parade, Kilkenny.
T 056 7786927

The Designer Exchange Swap Shop
Unit 1 Primose Forge, Hazelhatch
Road, Celbridge, Co. Kildare.
T 01 6544358
www.thedesignerexchange.net

Tiger Lily Boutique
Oliver Plunkett Street, Oldcastle,
Co. Meath. T 049 8550818

Toil and Glitter
5 Theatre Lane, Greystones,
Co. Wicklow. T 01 2017426
www.toilandglitter.com

Tuchuzy
Church Road, Greystones, Co. Wicklow.
T 01 2557867

Unique Boutique
39 Pearse Street, Mullingar,
Co. Westmeath. T 044 9341341

Utopia Boutique
Market Place, Main Street,
Dunshaughlin, Co. Meath. T 01 8258844

Vanity Fair
Unit 3, The Courtyard Shopping Centre,
Newbridge, Co. Kildare. T 045 431905

Vigi
Abbey Street, Wicklow. T 0404 10656

Wardrobe
Fitzwilliam Square, Wicklow.
T 0404 68649

Independent boutiques
Munster

Anna's
Tramway Terrace, Douglas Village,
Cork. T 021 4362231

Bamboo
The Cottage, Ardfert Village, Tralee,
Co. Kerry. T 066 7115915

Bella Sola
4 Bishop Street, Newcastlewest,
Co. Limerick. T 069 78222

Beth
17 French Church Street, Cork.
T 021 4274300
www.bouevardbeth.com

Cali Womenswear
Broderick Street, Midleton, Co. Cork.
T 021 4631999

Coco
41 William Street, Listowel, Co. Kerry.
T 068 23069

Cocoon
6 Emmet Place, Cork. T 021 4273393

Corcra
The Buttermarket, Market Street,
Clonmel, Co. Tipperary. T 052 87336
www.corcra.com

Designer Fusion
Winthrop Arcade, Winthorp Street,
Co. Cork. T 021 4270211

The Dressing Room
4 Emmet Place, Cork. T 021 4270117

Ealu
15 Percival Street, Kanturk, Co. Cork.
T 029 20866

Edel's Boutique
Friar Street, Nenagh, Co. Tipperary.
T 067 43186
www.edelsboutique.com

Effigy
14 Russell Street, Tralee, Co. Kerry.
T 066 7120938

Ela Maria
· The Square House, Newcastlewest,
  Co. Limerick. T 069 62855
· 2 Salt House Lane, Ennis, Co. Clare.
  T 065 6842873
· 9 Rock Street, Tralee, Co. Kerry.
  T 066 7123230
www.elamaria.com

Envy Boutique
50 New Street, Killarney, Co. Kerry.
T 064 6622072
www.envyboutique.ie

Flax in Bloom
Crusies Street, Limerick. T 061 318891

Footsteps
· Croke Street, Thurles, Co. Tipperary.
  T 0504 26747
· 54 Main Street, Tipperary. T 062 31653
www.footstepsshoes.ie

Gooseberry
· 43 Ashe Street, Clonakilty, Co. Cork.
  T 023 35812
· 35 North Street, Skibbereen,
  West Cork. T 028 23885

Inka
14b French Church Street, Co. Cork.
T 021 4254929

Iota
1 Mary Street, Tralee, Co. Kerry.
T 066 7129465

Joanne's Fashion House
Ballina, Killaloe, Co. Clare. T 061 375735

JR's
· 53 Thomas Street, Co. Limerick.
  T 061 408866
· 10 Kenyon Street, Nenagh,
  Co. Tipperary. T 067 33266

Katie Jane's
Castletroy Shopping Centre,
Castletroy, Limerick. T 061 333739

Katwalk Boutique
Collbawn, Broderick Street, Midleton,
Co. Cork. T 021 4613036

Kelly's
75–76 The Quay, Waterford. T 051 873557

Kimono
· North Quay, Newcastlewest,
  Co. Limerick. T 069 78820
· Main Street, Charleville, Co. Cork.
  T 063 21602
www.kimono.ie

La Boheme
Green Street, Dingle, Co. Kerry.
T 066 9152444

La Mode
74a O'Connell Street, Dungarvan,
Co. Waterford. T 058 43375

Le Chateau
Liberty Square, Thurles, Co. Tipperary.
T 0504 26535

Lily & Clara
· Unit 11 Time Square, Ballincollig,
  Co. Cork. T 021 4870424
· 139 Bank Place, Mallow, Co. Cork.
  T 022 51819
www.lilyandclara.ie

Luca
30 Princes Street, Cork.
T 021 4270440

Macbees
25 New Street, Killarney, Co. Kerry.
T 064 33622
www.macbees.ie

Marie Therese
4 The Mall, Thurles, Co. Tipperary.
T 0504 26791

Miriam Halley's Boutique
Main Guard, 57 Gladstone Street,
Clonmel, Co. Tipperary. T 052 27444

Moda
143 Main Street, Mallow, Co. Cork.
T 022 42737

Monica John
· 13/14 French Church Street, Cork.
  T 021 4271399
· High Street, Bantry, Co. Cork.
  T 027 51355

Muse
92 The Quay, Waterford. T 051 854448

Naphisa Boutique
1st Floor, 4 Cook Street, Cork.
T 021 4273787

Nelo Maternity
53 Roches Street, Co. Limerick.
T 061 207146
www.nelomaternity.com

Noa Noa
26 Oliver Plunkett Street, Cork.
T 021 4222727

Nozomi
· 60 Catherine Street, Limerick.
  T 061 467408
· 71 O'Connell Street, Ennis, Clare.
  T 065 6828655
www.nozomiennis.com

O'Dwyer Footwear
· 65 Main Street, Midleton, Co. Cork.
  T 021 4631572
· 114 Oliver Plunkett Street, Cork.
  T 021 4273949
· 84 North Main Street, Youghal,
  Co. Cork. T 024 90006
· The Bridge Shopping Centre,
  Dungarvan, Co. Waterford.
  T 058 24806

Opera on the Square
Fethard, Co. Tipperary. T 052 32659

Orchid Boutique
Unit 1 Ballinakill Shopping Centre,
Dunmore Road, Waterford.
T 051 859360

Paperdolls
3 Little Catherine Street, Limerick.
T 061 449956

The People of Oslo
George's Court, George's Street,
Waterford. T 051 844850

Perfect Paris
10 Church Street, Listowel Co. Kerry.
T 068 23773

Platform Boutique
Bridewell Row, Newcastlewest,
Co. Limerick. T 069 786147

Ruby
1 Ivy Terrace, Tralee, Co. Kerry.
T 066 7117796
www.ruby.ie

Satina
Queen Street, Tramore, Co. Waterford.
T 051 386600

Scalazell
98-99 Main Street, Cashel,
Co. Tipperary. T 062 64857

Scarlet Ribbon
Chapel Place, New Street, Killarney,
Co. Kerry. T 062 30003

Serenity
6 Main Street, Listowel, Co. Kerry.
T 068 24319
www.serenityfashions.com

Sheena's Boutique
• 24 Oliver Plunkett Street, Cork.
  T 021 4270574
• 85 Main Street, Midleton, Co. Cork.
www.sheenas.ie

Shoe Flair
• 56 Roches Street, Limerick.
  T 061 318686
• Mitchell Street, Nenagh,
  Co. Tipperary. T 067 37536
• Market Street, Ennis, Co. Clare.
  T 065 6893741
• Bridge Street, Newcastlewest,
  Co. Limerick. T 069 77755

Shoe La La
11 Ballinakill Shopping Centre,
Dunmore Road, Waterford. T 051 854963

Shoebaloo
94 The Quay, Waterford. T 051 871472
www.shoebaloo.net

Sinead's Boutique
Salmon Weir, Annacotty, Co. Limerick.
T 061 339696

South Beach
70 Main Street, Youghal, Co. Cork.
T 024 90943

The Style Room
36 New Street, Killarney, Co. Kerry.
T 064 39252

Sugar
Shearwater Pier Road, Kinsale, Co. Cork.
T 021 4774849

Sweetie P's Boutique
Royal Parade House, Killaloe, Co. Clare.
T 061 662685
www.sweetieps.ie

Taelane Boutique
Tae Lane, Listowel, Co. Kerry.
T 068 53885

Tippe Canoe
The Old Cornstore, Shannon Street,
Limerick. T 061 444804

The Warehouse Clonmel
37 Gladstone Street, Clonmel,
Co. Tipperary. T 052 6126922

Whisper Boutique
Ivy Terrace, Tralee, Co. Kerry.
T 066 7120020

Wild Pair
Ivy Terrace, Tralee, Co. Kerry.
T 066 7185675

Willow
4 O'Connell Street, Ennis, Co. Clare.
T 065 6891342

Wow
1 Mary Street, Tralee, Co. Kerry.
T 066 7117684

Independent boutiques
Belfast

Atelier
31 Queens Arcade, Belfast.
T 028 90278008

Brazil
Wellington Place and Bradbury Place,
Belfast. T 028 90245552

Carter
• 11 Upper Queen Street, Belfast.
  T 028 90243412
• 555 Lisburn Road, Belfast.
  T 028 90669335
www.carter-clothing.com

Cruise
Victoria Square, Belfast.
T 028 90320550
www.cruiseclothing.co.uk

Harpers
Lesley Plaza, 406 Lisburn Road, Belfast.
T 028 90681556
www.haperbelfast.com

Honey
627 Lisburn Road, Belfast.
T 028 90667466
www.honeycollection.co.uk

Nine Chichester Street
9 Chichester Street, Belfast.
T 028 90233308
www.ninechichesterstreet.com

Rojo Shoes
613 Lisburn Road, Belfast.
T 028 90666998
www.rojoshoes.co.uk

Roxbury & McQueen
473 Lisburn Road, Belfast.
T 028 90681332
www.roxburyandmcqueen.com

Statement at Margaret Giboney
527 Lisburn Road, Belfast.
T 028 90664507

The Velvet Boutique
661 Lisburn Road, Belfast.
T 028 90665221

The White Bicycle
50 Bloomfield Avenue, Belfast.
T 028 90457719
www.thewhitebicycle.co.uk

Una Roden Couture
50 Upper Arthur Street, Belfast.
T 028 90248811

Outlet Villages

Kildare Village
Nurney Road, Kildare.
T 045 520501
www.kildarevillage.com

Junction One
Antrim, BT414 LL.
T 0505 48900
www.junctionone.co.uk

Rathdowney Shopping Outlet
Rathdowney, Co. Laois.
T 0505 48900
www.rathdowneyoutlet.ie

The Outlet
Bridgewater Park, Banbridge,
BT32 4GJ.
T 028 40625151
www.the-outlet.co.uk

Some of Sonya and Brendan's favourite websites

www.asos.com
Look like your favourite celebrity from screen or stage!

www.fifibelle.com
Beautiful larger shoes

www.pretty-small-shoes.com
Exactly what it says on the tin!

www.my-wardrobe.com

www.littlewoodsireland.ie
Great for bigger girls!

www.style.com
Check out the latest from the catwalks to stay one step ahead of the posse.

www.yoox.com
Thousands of products with a wide range of prices.

www.net-a-porter.com
High-end fashion at high-end prices. Great eye candy!

www.jaeger.co.uk
Great classic essential elements.

www.isabellaoliver.com
Fab maternity wear, and, more recently, non-maternity wear.

www.apc.fr
Classic French youth chic.

www.toast.co.uk

www.mytights.com
Hosiery in every colour and style.

www.topshop.com
Fabulous interactive site from the king of the chain stores.

www.figleaves.co.uk
Comprehensive lingerie and swimwear specialist.

www.bravissimo.com

Disclaimer: The authors have made every reasonable effort to provide the most up to date details for the information contained in this shopping guide.

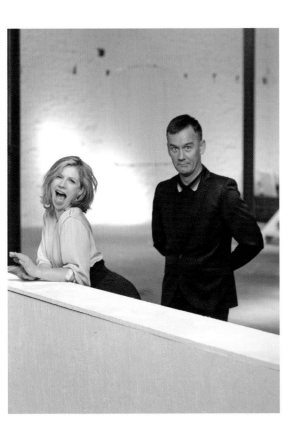

We hope that you've enjoyed the OFF THE RAILS: Love Your Look journey. Please remember that the advice, tips and guidelines we offer are all suggestions. You can do as much or as little as you are comfortable with – the real transformation begins with you.

We've helped you to identify your body shape, find the right underwear, and look at your body with a fresh and more appreciative eye. We've guided you towards the styles that will flatter your shape and get you noticed, and we've encouraged you to get a style buddy to support you on your mission. Now it's over to you – go ahead and knock 'em dead!

We hope you feel you've gained something from reading this book. We had great fun putting it together, and want you to have fun with it too. *Sonya & Brendan*

Leabharlanna Poibli Chathair Bhaile Átha Cliath
Dublin City Public Libraries

Acknowledgements

All our fabulous ladies who let us into their lives and inspired us to write this book. Our gorgeous son, Colm Corrigan. Sinéad O'Connor, Aifric Ní Chianáin and all the brilliant team on OFF THE RAILS – we love you! RTÉ's finest – Mary Curtis, Grainne McAleer and Niamh Farren. Christine Lucignano – make-up goddess. Zara Cox – the ultimate hair messer, and all the dudes at Queen Beauty Emporium. Clodagh Weber – 'knicker picker' extraordinaire. Kip Carroll and his fantastic assistant Trevor Darcy – for being the best and fastest triggers in town – great pics boys! All our fabulous contributors, including Derrick Carberry, Ken Boylan and Noel Sutton. David Smith and Oran Day at Atelier – design supremos. Chenile Keogh and Robert Doran at Merlin Publishing for their enthusiasm and unwavering support. Síne Quinn – our tireless editor and mind reader. Kate O Hora – told you I would. Our gorgeous friends and families for their love and support always, XXX. The wonderful world of fashion retail – we salute you!

Stockists for photo shoot:

Arnotts	Marks & Spencer
Coast	Oasis
Costume	River Island
Debenhams	Sabotage
Dunnes Stores	Topshop
Fitzpatrick Shoes	United Colors
Fran & Jane	of Benetton
House of Fraser	Wallis
Karen Millen	Warehouse